Epilepsy

A Handbook for the Mental Health Professional

Epilepsy

A Handbook for the Mental Health Professional

Edited by

Harry Sands, Ph.D.
Executive Director and
Director of Research,
Postgraduate Center for
Mental Health, New York

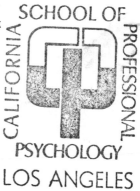

BRUNNER/MAZEL, Publishers • New York

Library of Congress Cataloging in Publication Data

Main entry under title:

Epilepsy, a handbook for the mental health
professional.

   Bibliography: p
   Includes index.
   1. Epilepsy—Handbooks, manuals, etc.
2. Epilepsy—Psychological aspects—Handbooks,
manuals, etc. 3. Psychotherapy—Handbooks,
manuals, etc. I. Sands, Harry.
RC372.E658   616.8'53   81-12237
ISBN 0-87630-272-X   AACR2

Published by
BRUNNER/MAZEL, INC.
19 Union Square
New York, New York 10003

To my wife Helene and sons Jeff and Rick.

CONTENTS

IV. HELPING RESOURCES

ACKNOWLEDGMENTS

First and foremost, I wish to thank the Esther A. and Joseph Klingenstein Fund, Inc., for its generous help in the preparation of this book and of the larger project, including a training program in epilepsy for mental health professionals, of which the book forms a part. I especially thank John Klingenstein for his personal support and encouragement.

Dr. William Young's research was instrumental in securing the data base that identified the information which those in the field of mental health need if they are to help persons with epilepsy. Providing this information became the goal of this book.

Dr. Richard L. Masland, former Director of the Commission for the Control of Epilepsy and Its Consequences and H. Houston Merritt Professor of Neurology, College of Physicians and Surgeons, Columbia University, gave us ongoing advice based on his extensive knowledge of the many aspects of the epilepsies and was a constant source of encouragment and help. Dr. Lewis R. Wolberg, Director Emeritus of the Postgraduate Center for Mental Health and Clinical Professor of Psychiatry, New York University School of Medicine, from the outset guided us in meeting our goal of supplying information that would enable mental health practitioners to provide treatment for the psychological and social problems associated with epilepsy.

The enthusiastic cooperation of all the contributors brought excitement and pleasure to the task, and Ms. Frances C. Minters' executive abilities and editorial management skills assured that the pieces would come together and achieve their purpose.

I thank all of these wonderful people for helping make this book a reality.

INTRODUCTION

Epileptologists generally agree that persons with epilepsy show a relatively high frequency of emotional disturbances and adjustment problems. Thus Rodin et al.[1] report that 54 percent of epilepsy patients have such problems, while Blumer[2] asserts that between one-sixth and one-quarter of outpatients with epilepsy have psychiatric disorders, and Dodrill concludes that emotional problems are in the forefront of patients' adjustment difficulties (see Chapter 5, this volume).

A wide range of psychopathology has also been reported, running the gamut from the psychoses through character disorders, chronic depressions, and anxiety neuroses.[3,4] Similarly, the incidence of psychiatric disorders among children with epilepsy has been found to be four times higher than in children in the general population. Indeed, emotional and adjustment problems are so widespread that the Commission for the Control of Epilepsy and Its Consequences asserts, "The social, psychological, and behavioral problems that frequently accompany epilepsy can be more handicapping than the actual seizures."[5]

The mental health practitioner who is called upon to help a person with epilepsy deal with these psychological and social concomitants of his or her disorder is faced with a complex of determinants idiosyncratic to epilepsy. Central to assessing these psychosocial problems and to developing a psychological treatment strategy is the clinician's understanding of the neurological, neurobiological, and neuropsychological, as well as social, ethnic and economic, factors associated with epilepsy.

Focus on Understanding Seizure Mechanisms

In the first book about epilepsy, *On the Sacred Disease*, written about 400 B.C., Hippocrates noted that epilepsy was due to a disturbance in the brain.[6] This truth was largely ignored for centuries, while physicians used supernatural means to explain epilepsy. The brain's role in epilepsy again became important in the mid-nineteenth century, when Hughlings Jackson, the founder of modern neurology, focused on the brain as the organ involved in epilepsy.[7] From that time to the present, an all-out effort in epilepsy research was made to gain an understanding of the neural mechanisms of seizures and the control of seizures with anticonvulsants.

Since the brain is also the center of the human psyche, one would have expected a concurrent interest in the psychological or the behavioral aspects of epilepsy. This, however, was not the case. The ongoing attention was to epilepsy's dramatic symptom, seizures, while the other factors—psychological and social—have drawn little interest. Indeed, according to the Commission for the Control of Epilepsy and Its Consequences, despite their common occurrence they have been "the most neglected aspect of epilepsy."[8]

FOCUS ON PSYCHOLOGICAL AND SOCIAL FACTORS

Epilepsy, for the most part, has been the domain of neurology; psychiatry's concern was almost exclusively with the seizure patients who had psychoses, or who were institutionalized in state hospitals and epilepsy colonies.[9] Several factors, however, have now combined to change that emphasis.

First, antiepileptic drugs can now successfully control seizures—the major symptom of epilepsy—for most patients with epilepsy. Then, the current interest in treating the "whole person" has brought with it a concern for dealing with psychosocial problems. This is also an outcome of the citizens' movement, such as the Epilepsy Foundation of America. The citizens' movement in epilepsy has emphasized *all* the needs of people with epilepsy, and particularly the psychological and social needs. The rehabilitation-of-the-handicapped field has also helped, with its focus on psychosocial factors which interfere with the disabled person's ability to work, to adjust to the tasks of daily living, and to live independently in the community. A further impetus to change has come from the patients' rights movement.

Additional interest in the psychological and social factors comes from their role as triggers of seizures and their use in psychological treatment—in conjunction with the antiepileptic drugs—for the control of seizures [10] (also see Chapter 2, this volume), as well as from recognition that the patient's attitude and motivation play an essential role in clinical management program. For example, Feldman and Ricks state:

> The epileptic patient must be able to accept the diagnosis and the various psychological and social ramifications that accompany it. For an epileptic to be willing to take medicine every day, tolerate occasional side effects, and still run the risk of having another seizure, he must be provided with information that will enable him to believe he has some degree of control over what happens to him.[11]

Thus, the emphasis has now expanded to include the psychological and social problems of epilepsy. The epileptologist's acceptance that the patient's behavior and attitudes play a significant role in achieving seizure control and effective coping with the tasks of daily living makes the full range of individual and family counseling and psychotherapy an integral part of the clinical management of the patient with epilepsy. Accordingly, counseling, which includes providing information and education about epilepsy and psychotherapy directed at changing behavior patterns, should start at the time the diagnosis of epilepsy is made, and should be administered concurrently with the anticonvulsant drugs in keeping with the patient's and family's needs.

FOCUS ON INFORMATION

Little information about epilepsy is given in medical schools or graduate schools of psychology, social work, or counseling training programs. All mental health clinicians require more knowledge about epilepsy in order that they may use their therapeutic skills and resources to deal with the psychological and social problems of persons with epilepsy. This is borne out in a national survey of 749 mental health administrators and mental health facilities (Table 1).[12] In response to a questionnaire, 59 percent stated that they would be interested in extending services to patients with epilepsy. Sixty-eight percent indicated a need for sociological/psychological information; 41 percent for didactic knowledge—symptomatology, treatment procedures, and neuropsychiatric information; 40 percent for medical/physiological implications for intervention; and 34 percent for diagnosis, especially differentiating psychological/physiological (Table 2).

The results of this study serve, in part, as the basis for the selection of topics and materials for inclusion in this book. The purpose of this book is to provide necessary information about epilepsy to the core mental health disciplines: psychiatry, psychology, social work, and psychiatric nursing; and to other, collaborating disciplines, such as rehabilitation and counseling. The information is intended to enable these practitioners to counsel and treat the complex psychological and social problems so that the person with epilepsy will gain maximum fulfillment and actualization of his or her abilities, and independence in the community.

Accordingly, in Chapter 1, Dr. Masland deals with the neurology of seizures, diagnosis, and treatment, including antiepileptic drugs and their side effects and interactions. In Chapter 2, Dr. Williams discusses conditioned response procedures, hypnosis, biofeedback and desensitization as adjunctive to the antiepileptic drugs. In Chapter 3, Dr. Sherwin covers behavior

Table 1

Survey of Mental Health Administrators and Facilities

Facility	Number
State and Regional Mental Health Administrators	53
CMHC's (Federally funded Community Mental Health Centers)	478
Public Mental Health Centers	143
Private Mental Hospitals	48
VA Outpatient Psychiatric Clinics	27
Total	749

Source: Sands & Young, 1978

Table 2

Survey of Mental Health Administrators and Facilities

Question No. 12: What is important for your staff to know?

	Percent
A) Sociological/psychosocial	68
B) Correct misinformation and/or present bad practice	12
C) Medication/physiological implications to intervention	40
D) Staff skills in teaching epileptics to live with their handicap—management guidelines	25
E) Didactic knowledge: Symptomatology, treatment procedures, neuropsychiatric	41
F) Recent advances	5
G) Law	3
H) Diagnosis, especially differentiating psychological/physiological	34
I) Community programs/vocational	12
J) Emergency procedures—safeguard procedures	16

Source: Sands & Young, 1978

arising from the various ictal (seizure) conditions, the anticonvulsant drugs, and the architectural structures of the brain; the ictal disturbances arising from temporal lobe epilepsy (partial seizures) are included here. In Chapter 4, Dr. Blumer focuses on the treatment of specific psychiatric complications of institutional patients with epilepsy. In Chapter 5, Dr. Dodrill focuses on special neuropsychological tests designed to assess cognitive functions and to measure levels of personal adjustment in persons with seizure disorders.

The psychotherapy section begins with Chapter 6, in which Dr. Sands presents the psychodynamic method for understanding neurological, psychological, social and economic factors in determining behavior of patients with epilepsy and the considerations for conducting dynamic short-term therapy. In Chapter 7, Dr. Ziegler discusses psychotherapy and counseling for the child with epilepsy and his or her family.

In Chapter 8, Drs. Fraser and Smith discuss helping patients with reactive problems, daily living skills, and interpersonal relationships. Finally, in Chapter 9, Dr. Levinson provides information and referral resources—lists of federal, state, local, and voluntary services and aid—available for persons with epilepsy and their families.

This information is designed to give a data base for the clinical management of persons with epilepsy, and to enable mental health practitioners to deal with the multivaried problems which patients present.

HARRY SANDS, PH.D.
Walter Mill, N.Y.

REFERENCES

1. Rodin, E. A., Shapiro, H. L., and Lennox, K.: Epilepsy and life performance. *Rehabilitation Literature* 38:34-39, 1977.
2. Blumer, D.: Temporal Lobe Epilepsy and Its Psychiatric Significance. Commission for the Control of Epilepsy and Its Consequences, Vol. II, Part 1, p. 359. U.S. Department of Health, Education, and Welfare, Public Health Service, National Institute of Health, DHEW, Publication No. (NIH) 78-276, 1978.
3. Stevens, J. R.: Psychiatric implications of psychomotor epilepsy. *Arch. Gen. Psychiat.* 14:461-471, 1966.
4. Price-Phillips, W.: Psychiatric and Psychological Aspects of Epilepsy. Commission for the Control of Epilepsy and Its Consequences, Vol. II, Part 1, p. 361. U.S. Department of Health, Education, and Welfare, Public Health Service, National Institute of Health, DHEW, Publication No. (NIH) 78-276, 1978.
5. Commission for the Control of Epilepsy and Its Consequences; Plan for Nationwide Action on Epilepsy, Vol. I, Social Adjustment and Mental Health, p. 73, 1978.
6. Temkin, O.: *The Falling Sickness.* Baltimore: The Johns Hopkins Press, 1945.
7. Taylor, J. (ed.): *Selected Writings of John Hughlings Jackson,* Vol. I, *On Epilepsy and Epileptiform Convulsions.* New York: Basic Books, 1931, p. 500.

8. Commission for the Control of Epilepsy, op. cit., p. 35.
9. Sands, H.: Statement to the Commission for the Control of Epilepsy and Its Consequences, Vol. II, Part I, p. 363. U.S. Department of Health, Education, and Welfare, Public Health Service, National Institute of Health, DHEW, Publication No. (NIH) 78-276.
10. Feldman, R. G. and Ricks, N. L.: Nonpharmacological and behavioral methods, Chapter XI, 89-125. In: Ferris, G. S. (ed.), *Treatment of Epilepsy Today*. Oradell, N.J.: Medical Economics Co., Book Division, 1978, pp. 218.
11. Ibid, p. 89.
12. Sands, H., and Young, W.: An evaluation of the status of epilepsy in the mental health system. Proceedings 10th International Epilepsy Symposium, Vancouver, B.C., September 10, 1978.

CONTRIBUTORS

DIETRICH BLUMER, M.D.
Chairman, Department of Psychiatry, Henry Ford Hospital; Clinical Professor of Psychiatry, University of Michigan, Detroit, Michigan

CARL B. DODRILL, Ph.D.
Associate Professor of Neurological Surgery, School of Medicine, University of Washington, Seattle, Washington

ROBERT T. FRASER, Ph.D.
Director, Vocational Service, Epilepsy Center; Research Assistant Professor, Departments of Neurosurgery and Rehabilitation Medicine, University of Washington, Seattle, Washington

RISHA W. LEVINSON, D.S.W.
Associate Professor of Social Policy, Adelphi University. School of Social Work, Garden City, New York

RICHARD L. MASLAND, M.D.
H. Houston Merritt Professor of Neurology Emeritus, College of Physicians and Surgeons, Columbia University, New York

HARRY SANDS, Ph.D.
Executive Director, Postgraduate Center for Mental Health, New York, New York

IRA SHERWIN, M.D.
Associate Chief of Staff, Research and Development, E.N.R.M. V.A. Hospital and Department of Neurology, Harvard University, Cambridge, Massachusetts

WAYNE R. SMITH, Ph.D.
Research Associate, Sexual Assault Center, University of Washington, Seattle, Washington

DANIEL T. WILLIAMS, M.D.
Assistant Professor of Clinical Psychiatry, Director of the Pediatric Neuropsychiatry Service, Columbia Presbyterian Medical Center, New York

ROBERT G. ZIEGLER, M.D.
Director, Family Service Team, Seizure Unit, Departments of Psychiatry and Neurology, Children's Hospital Medical Center, Boston, Massachusetts

Epilepsy
A Handbook for the Mental Health Professional

I.
THE NATURE AND TREATMENT OF EPILEPSY

1

THE NATURE OF EPILEPSY

RICHARD L. MASLAND, M.D.

The essential feature of an epileptic seizure is the occurrence of a paroxysm of synchronized overactivity of a group of nerve cells within the brain. This overactivity may be recorded by the use of electroencephalogram (EEG) or by more direct means for measuring the electrical activity of the brain. It is commonly manifested by a concomitant paroxysmal change in behavior—that is, change in cognitive function, sensation, or movement.

By arbitrary definition, a person is said to "have epilepsy" when he or she has experienced two or more epileptic seizures in the absence of an evident precipitating factor such as fever, infection, metabolic disease, or toxin (such as alcohol).[1] Probably persons who have had a single epileptic seizure, who have abnormal EEG, but who have been prevented from exhibiting additional seizures by the use of anticonvulsant drugs should also be considered epileptic.

CAUSES OF EPILEPSY

There are many different causes of epileptic seizures. A number of "animal models"—experimentally induced seizures—have provided valuable clues as to the various mechanisms whereby seizures may be produced.

Seizures of Local Origin

Appropriate stimulation of a group of nerve cells of the cerebrum can cause these cells to develop a paroxysm of overactivity. If this activity reaches a sufficient amplitude, it may spread throughout the nervous system. If the excitation remains limited to its site of origin, it is spoken of as a *partial* (*local* or *focal*) *seizure*. If it spreads, it is said to have produced a *secondary generalized seizure*. Focal seizures may be generated in animals by rhythm-

5

ical electrical stimulation, local application of chemicals, or local injury and scar formation.

Rhythmic Electrical Stimulation. When nerve cells are stimulated with repetitive electrical stimuli, they fall into step with this stimulation, and a repetitive synchronous discharge results. If an adequate stimulus is continued for more than a few seconds, a focal seizure is produced, and this may spread to become generalized.

It is of particular interest that the occurrence of such an episode must have some long-lasting facilitating effect on the brain. With each subsequent stimulation, the strength and duration of the adequate stimulus are reduced, and the tendency to spread is increased. This phenomenon is termed *kindling.* In certain animals, daily stimulation of the brain for periods of only 30 seconds, if repeated over a period of months, will ultimately lead to such a level of brain overexcitability as to be associated with abnormalities of the EEG between seizures and even spontaneous epileptic seizures. Spread of abnormal excitability to other parts of the brain far removed from the site of the stimulus can also be demonstrated.[2]

Local Application of Chemicals. Stimulant drugs such as picrotoxin, cardiazol (Metrazol), acetyl choline, or penicillin, if applied locally to the brain, will produce partial seizures just as does electrical stimulation. Some of these agents clearly act by manipulation of excitatory and inhibitory neurotransmitters and by alteration of the excitability cycles of the neurons. The result is to generate bursts of high frequency neuronal discharges superimposed on slow potential shifts within the nerve cell membranes. When these discharges become synchronized and reach a critical level, a propagated seizure occurs. As with electrical stimulation, repeated local injection of stimulant drugs leads to lowering of threshold and enhanced spread of the seizure discharge.[3]

Local Injury and Scar Formation. Freezing of an area of the brain will cause the damaged area to become epileptogenic for hours or even days after the insult. The injection into the brain of sclerosing agents, especially cobalt powder or aluminum hydroxide paste, may cause the animal to have recurrent partial epileptic seizures over a period of months or years. Excision of the focus leads to cessation of the seizures. The process whereby this state of chronic neuronal hyperexcitability is induced is not clearly understood. The fact that aluminum and cobalt are specifically effective suggests that there may be some biochemical effect. However, the fact that similar seizures occur in humans as a result of simple brain trauma suggests that it may be the scar-producing effects of these agents and their effect on the supporting elements of the brain, rather than a direct chemical effect on the neurons, that produces the seizure state. Experimental injection of blood or iron salts also produces an epileptic focus, suggesting another possible mechanism for human post-traumatic epilepsy, that is, intracerebral hemorrhage.[4]

Seizures with Factors Affecting the Entire Brain

Whereas the partial or focal seizures described above originate within a specific area and may or may not spread to involve the entire brain, other types of seizures appear to reflect a hyperexcitability or instability of the entire brain, or of neural systems within the brain. Such seizures are likely to be generalized from their onset, an entire network of brain cells being involved almost simultaneously in the hypersynchrony that is the hallmark of epilepsy. Generalized seizures may be produced by electrical stimulation, drugs, chemical agents, or genetic susceptibility. Generalized seizures may be caused by a variety of mechanisms.

Electrical Stimulation. Electrical stimulation of certain structures from which efferent pathways extend widely throughout the brain can produce seizures that have no local sign and that are generalized from the onset. The most striking are those resulting from stimulation of certain nuclei in the thalamic region of the brain which appear to serve a pacemaker or regulatory role on the cortex.

Drugs. Alteration of general neuronal excitability by drugs or chemicals can precipitate generalized seizures. Large intravenous doses of cardiazol (Metrazol), strychnine, or picrotoxin may have this effect. Tetanus produces not only peripheral and spinal hyperactivity, but centrally generated seizures as well.

Chemical Agents. Chemical agents which interfere with the inhibitory neurotransmitter Gamma amino butyric acid (GABA) cause generalized hyperactivity and lead to spontaneous seizures. Vitamin B6 deficiency, agene (a bleaching agent of flour), and bicuculline are examples of agents which produce seizures in man and animals by this mechanism.

Genetic Susceptibility. Genetic susceptibility plays an important part in the occurrence of seizures in various strains of animals. A number of strains of seizure-prone animals have been developed. In some instances, seizures are spontaneous;[5] in others, they are induced by visual or auditory stimulation. One strain of mice becomes susceptible to sound-produced seizures only if the mice experience a single brief exposure to a loud tone during a critical phase of early development. Certain epileptic baboons experience seizures when exposed to a flashing light, as do persons with photosensitive epilepsy.

TYPES OF EPILEPSY

In human beings, epilepsy is divided into two main classifications: partial and generalized (see Table 1).

The "Partial" Epilepsies (Focal or Local)

Any injury or disorder affecting a part of the brain may produce a scar or epileptic focus which subsequently serves as a trigger for epileptic seizures. The known causes of such epilepsies, also spoken of as "symptomatic," are shown in Table 2.

Symptomatic epilepsies are most commonly manifested by seizures of local onset—the first sign of the seizure reflecting activation of that part of the brain in which the focus is located—and in this event they are spoken of as *partial*. When the brain injury or disorder is a diffuse one, the subject may exhibit many different seizure types, and a condition called *secondary generalized* epilepsy may ensue (that is, generalized epilepsy secondary to brain disease).

Table 1

International Classification of the Epilepsies

   I. *Generalized Epilepsies*
      1. Primary generalized epilepsies (includes petit mal and grand mal seizures)
      2. Secondary generalized epilepsies
      3. Undetermined generalized epilepsies
  II. *Partial (focal, local) Epilepsies* (includes Jacksonian, temporal lobe, and psychomotor seizures)
 III. *Unclassifiable Epilepsies*

Table 2

Causes of Symptomatic Epilepsy in Patients
Undergoing Operations for Focal Epileptogenic Lesions

Perinatal	43.3%
Infection	26.7%
Trauma	16.7%
Tumor	5.0%
Unknown	3.3%
	100.0%

The "Primary Generalized" Epilepsies

In many instances of epilepsy there is no evident anatomic pathology, and the occurrence of seizures with their electrical concomitants is the sole manifestation of the underlying disorder. In such instances the seizures show no focal sign. They are generalized and bilateral in onset, the initial manifestation being loss of consciousness without aura. The primary generalized epilepsies often depend upon a constitutionally determined low seizure threshold, and genetic factors are especially prominent.

SPECIFIC FORMS OF EPILEPSY AND THEIR RELATED SEIZURE TYPES

The accepted classification of epileptic seizures is shown in Table 3. The types are explained below.

Table 3

International Classification of Epileptic Seizures

 I. *Partial Seizures* (seizures beginning locally)
   A. Partial seizures with elementary symptomatology (generally without impairment of consciousness)
      1. With motor symptoms (includes Jacksonian seizures)
      2. With special sensory or somatosensory symptoms
      3. With autonomic symptoms
      4. Compound forms
   B. Partial seizures with complex symptomatology (generally with impairment of consciousness)
      1. With impairment of consciousness only
      2. With cognitive symptomatology
      3. With affective symptomatology
      4. With "psychosensory" symptomatology
      5. With "psychomotor" symptomatology (automatisms)
      6. Compound forms
   C. Partial seizures secondarily generalized
 II. *Generalized Seizures* (bilaterally symmetrical and without local onset)
      1. Absences (petit mal)
      2. Bilateral massive epileptic myoclonus
      3. Infantile spasms
      4. Clonic seizures
      5. Tonic seizures
      6. Tonic-clonic seizures (grand mal)
      7. Atonic seizures
      8. Akinetic seizures
 III. *Unilateral Seizures* (or predominantly)
 IV. *Unclassified Epileptic Seizures* (due to incomplete data)

The Partial Epilepsies

The manifestations of partial epilepsy depend upon that part of the brain in which the focus of injury is located (Figure 1).

Partial Seizures with Elementary Symptomatology. Foci located in most areas of the frontal, parietal, and occipital lobe produce seizures whose initial symptoms represent elementary movement or sensation. From the sensory

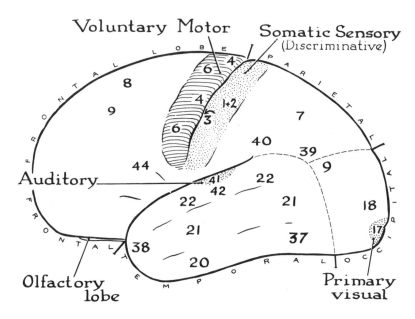

Figure 1. Diagram of left cerebral hemisphere numbered according to Brodmann's areas of the cortex. Electrical stimulation in conscious patients during surgical procedures has elicited the following responses:

Area 8: Head, eyes, trunk to the opposite side. Complex synergic movements of centralateral arm and leg.

Area 44: Arrest of speech.

Area 4 and 6: Stimulation of the lower end of the motor strip produces movement of face, tongue, jaw, palate and larynx. Above this is the thumb, thigh, digits and hand. At the upper end is the trunk, thigh, leg and foot.

Area 1, 2 and 3: Stimulation of the post central area produces sensations of tingling and numbness in area of the body corresponding to those of the adjacent motor strip.

Area 7: Disagreeable unlocalized sensations.

Area 9: Eyes to the opposite side.

Area 22 and 42: Acoustic hallucinations.

Area 21: Head, eyes, trunk to opposite side—complex synergic movements of centralateral extremities.

Area 18: Complex optic hallucinations.

motor area adjacent to the central sulcus arise seizures whose onset is with sensation or movement in a part of the body, spreading progressively to other areas—the classical *Jacksonian march*. Seizures originating in the parietal area start with a sensation as of a breeze blowing on the skin, or a light stroking sensation, tingling, or numbness; from this sensation comes the word *aura*, which in Greek means "breeze." Seizures from the precentral area start with rhythmical twitching of the face, arm, or leg. From the premotor area, the onset is with more complex movements—turning of head and eyes to the side, coordinated movements of the arm or trunk, or even turning of the whole body. With some focal frontal lobe epilepsies, loss of consciousness may occur at the onset, or may be the only symptom. Seizures originating in the occipital lobe begin with visual phenomena such as white or colored lights, balls, or other unformed objects.

Partial Seizures with Complex Symptomatology. Seizures originating in the temporal lobe (and occasionally inferior frontal) regions involve changes in cognition and behavior; that is, complex and coordinated thoughts or actions as opposed to elementary sensations or movements. These complex seizures have previously been termed *psychomotor*. The onset of a temporal lobe seizure may take any of the following forms:[6]

1. Subjective Symptoms
   a. *Elementary visceral sensations.* Peculiar (usually unpleasant) taste or odor, numbness of both hands, lips or tongue, choking and swallowing sensations.
   b. *Formed visual hallucinations.* The appearance before the eyes of a picture of a person or scene, familiar or unfamiliar. The same scene commonly recurs with repeated seizures.
   c. *Recollection of previous events or scenes.* Sudden recall of a scene or event. This phenomenon is closely related to the *déja vu* experience in which the individual experiences an overwhelming sense of familiarity—the feeling that he or she must have experienced or dreamed these circumstances before. This experience also is often as in a dream, which may or may not be recalled after the seizure.
   d. *Change in the appearance of surroundings.* Strangeness as opposed to familiarity; there may be a sense of strangeness or a feeling that other people's actions are odd. Things may have the Alice-in-Wonderland sensation of becoming larger or smaller, or of approaching or receding.
   e. *Change in emotions.* Sensations of terrible anxiety or dread, or of elation.
   f. *Aphasia.* Inability to comprehend and/or speak.

Note: Any of the above subjective symptoms may occur as the entire seizure, there being no outward indication; or they may progress to automatism or secondary generalized tonic-clonic seizure (see Table 4).

The following brief extracts from recorded interviews are presented to demonstrate the intangible quality of the subjective symptoms of persons suffering from complex partial seizures:

Headache: "My head starts hurting, and I start talking funny. Then, that's all I remember." "It just feels like something is coming through my head."

Numbness of Hand or Hands: "I have a tingle—I feel it coming in the end of my fingers and in my toes." "You know how your foot feels when it goes to sleep—It feels like that in my hands."

Lips, Mouth, Tongue, Throat: "It just feels like the top of my mouth drops down to the bottom." "The back of my mouth just swells."

Chest Pain or Restriction of Breathing: "There's something that chokes me. I can't get my breath."

Taste: "It was just a sour taste in my mouth—a burning sour taste, way in the back."

Nausea or Discomfort in Abdomen: "I had a funny feeling in the pit of my stomach as though things are going around and around."

Indescribable Feeling: "I feel as though I were out of gear—as though the blood had stopped circulating." "I sting all over for about a minute, and then I have a spell." "It's a queer feeling like a flash goes all through me. Sometimes it starts in my head and goes down."

Table 4

General Characteristics of Seizures

Combinations of seizure types observed in 40 patients with focal epileptic discharges (EEG) arising in the temporal region.

Type	Number
Generalized Convulsions Without Aura	9
Clinically Overt Minor Attacks and Convulsions	5
Clinically Overt Minor Attacks Only	1
Subjective Attacks, Clinically Overt Minor Attacks and Generalized Convulsions	17
Predominantly Subjective Minor Attacks Only	7
No Attacks	1
TOTAL	40

Déja Vu: "Maybe I'll be looking at something and maybe think like I had
   had a dream of something like I dreamt of being here before. Then the
   spell would come on." "It isn't that things seem closer. It's just that they
   seem so much more real. It is as though I had dreamed it before. If we
   were sitting here, it would be as if we had rehearsed this before, and I
   knew just exactly what you were going to say next."
Dream or Vision: "Sometimes I have thoughts of dreams. I can't remember
   what it was about, but at that time it's very vivid. One time I dreamed
   of the garden of Valhalla—it's things like that—just something out of this
   world."
   "I just had the feeling that everything was running together before me
   or something. I feel like I'm having a horrible illusion all of a sudden,
   and then the things in the room before me are the same, but I feel like
   I'm seeing scenes in a distance that I can't see clearly, or something like
   that." "All I know is that I just have a horrible feeling. I know I am having
   some sort of illusions, but I can never say what they are after it is over."
   "My mother had been dead three years. I saw my mother just as plain
   and lifelike figure as could ever be seen in this world. She threw up her
   hand and said, 'Come along son.' I hope no one ever experiences that
   feeling of seeing her there and knowing that she was dead."
Recollection: "I see some of my childhood scenes—just like a picture in front
   of my eyes. Most of them are just a flash."
Aphasia: "I might be talking on the telephone and suddenly I can't talk. I
   just sit there with the phone in my hand, and the person I am talking to
   says, 'Why don't you say something?'—I am that way for fifteen minutes
   sometimes."
Amnesia for Attack: "I was reading a book. I had laid it on the bed. The
   next thing I knew I was in the living room, and I didn't know where the
   book was."
   "I had a spell. I remembered putting the calves in. I was walking to
   the house and I looked down, and my shirt was muddy and my pants full
   of mud. I checked, and my horse must have dragged me fifty feet. I didn't
   even know that I had had an attack until I saw the mud on my feet."
Forced Thinking: "When things come into my mind I try to fight it, but still
   I have it." "If I can get my mind set on something, I can ward off the
   attack."

   The patterns of subjective aura observed in a series of patients with electroencephalographic evidences of temporal lobe epilepsy are summarized
in Table 5.

Table 5

Subjective Symptoms of 100 Persons with Temporal Lobe EEG Focus

Symptom	Number
Nausea or abdominal sensation	28
Faint or dizzy	27
Numbness of lips—choking	17
Headache	15
Inability to talk	15
Taste or smell	13
Dream state	12
Dread	12
Chest pain or inability to breathe	12
Funny feeling all over	11
Strange appearance of surroundings	10
Numbness of hands	10
Indescribable sensation	10
Vision	9
Palpitation	6
Déja vu	4
Recollection	3
Forced thinking	3
Auditory disturbance	1

2. Automatisms

Automatisms refer to loss of consciousness with automatic behavior. Unconsciousness may occur as the onset of the attack—the person losing consciousness without warning—or it may be preceded by subjective sensation. The automatism frequently starts with a brief arrest of activities, sometimes with chewing, swallowing, or salivation. There may be repetitive movements of the hands or shuffling of the feet. Automatic behavior varies from uncoordinated movements of the extremities to very complex activities, at times appearing normal but inappropriate. Attacks may last for up to fifteen minutes. Even brief episodes may be followed by amnesia and confusion. Violent behavior is uncommon; however, if attempts are made forcibly to control or hold the subject, a violent reaction may ensue.

The Primary Generalized Epilepsies

With Absence Seizures. Primary generalized epilepsy (PGE) with simple absence (commonly called *true petit mal*) usually starts between the ages of two and fifteen. It is characterized by brief lapses of consciousness *without aura.* During the attack there may be slight rhythmic movements of the eyelids and hands. An attack may be followed by a brief, poorly organized automatism. The attacks commonly last less than one or two minutes, and they are followed by rapid return to full consciousness without retrograde amnesia (although the person has no memory of what occurred during the period of the attack) or confusion. The EEG shows a characteristic pattern of paroxysms of 3-4/second spikes and waves, commonly precipitated by overbreathing. Absence seizures may or may not occur as the only manifestation of epilepsy.

With Tonic-Clonic Seizures. The tonic-clonic (*grand mal*) seizures of primary generalized epilepsy are generalized from the onset. The subject has no warning. The body suddenly becomes rigid with fully extended extremities and the breath is expelled, producing a cry. After a brief tonic (rigid) phase, the body begins to jerk. The jerks become slower and more gross. After two to ten minutes, the jerking ceases. The individual regains consciousness—usually confused, exhausted, and sleepy. The EEG between attacks may show bilateral spike-wave patterns, or it may be characterized by episodes of rapid fast sharp wave discharges. The attack is characterized by a momentary "flattening" of the record, followed by low voltage fast sharp waves.

Absence seizures and tonic-clonic seizures are two manifestations of primary generalized epilepsy that are closely related. They may occur independently, but they are frequently associated. Quite often, the disorder starts as absence only, then grand mal attacks occur. With adolescence, the absence attacks are more likely to stop than are the grand mal.

With Myoclonic and/or Akinetic Seizures. An important and little recognized form of epilepsy is that occurring during late childhood and adolescence and characterized by myoclonic and tonic-clonic seizures.[7] Subjects with such seizures are inclined to be nervous and high strung. They have difficulty in getting to sleep at night and are hard to wake in the morning. For the first hour or so after awakening (especially if awakened early and with difficulty), they are subject to repetitive symmetrical brief jerks. The arms are flexed and the trunk jerked forward. The jerks are so brief that lapse of consciousness is not evident. However, occasionally the jerks become rapidly repetitive and fused into a generalized clonic seizure. This form of epilepsy appears to have a different pathophysiology and genetic background from the absence and tonic-clonic epilepsies described above. The EEG also shows a different pattern, often associated with brief bursts of multiple spike-wave discharges synchronous with the myoclonus of the body.

The Photosensitive Epilepsies. In some individuals, seizures may be precipitated by a rhythmically flashing light; in others, specific visually presented patterns—grids, squares, or lines—may serve to precipitate an attack.

Attacks may be myoclonic in onset, as described above. Patients with photosensitive epilepsy may be genetically distinct and have different EEG characteristics from those who have the other forms of primary generalized epilepsy.

Benign Centrotemporal Paroxysms. A recently recognized form of epilepsy is that characterized by diurnal focal sensorimotor seizures with head-turning, and focal or generalized seizures during sleep. The EEG is characterized by focal epileptic spike discharges in the central (Rolandic) region of the brain. It is strikingly age-limited, appearing after age three and ceasing by age 15, with peak frequency at ages four to nine.

There is a strong family history in such seizures. They are unassociated with brain damage. The seizures disappear during adolescence in 50 percent of cases.[8]

The Secondary Generalized Epilepsies

A number of brain diseases that produce widespread neuronal damage lead to severe and uncontrollable seizures, characterized by their diversity within a given individual. Some, such as tuberous sclerosis in infancy and subacute sclerosing panencephalitis (SSPE) and Unverricht myoclonus in adults, are well recognized genetic or viral diseases. In others, the etiology is unknown, and even the pathology may be doubtful. The prognosis for these latter forms may be more favorable, and possibly some should be considered among the primary generalized epilepsies. Yet, in general, their malignant course and frequent association with severe mental retardation sets them apart. They are manifested by complex absence, myoclonic, astatic, akinetic, and tonic seizures. The seizure manifestations vary with the age of the patient, the seizures tending to become less frequent but more generalized and severe with increasing age.

Infantile Spasms. With infantile spasms, seizures almost always begin prior to age one, and never after age two. Seizures are frequently unrecognized in infancy because of their brief, shock-like character, easily mistaken for startle reaction. The child may give a sharp cry, accompanying it by shock-like extension of the trunk and arms. These brief jerks may occur every few minutes throughout the day, often in rapid series. As the infant ages, other types of seizures develop. The EEG shows gross abnormality with slow spike and wave patterns which may become almost continuous—the so-called hypsarrhythmia.

Myoclonic Astatic Epilepsy (Lennox-Gastaut). The Lennox-Gastaut syndrome may evolve from infantile spasms or may develop de novo in children after age two. It is also characterized by the diversity of its manifestations. The most common seizure is a *complex absence.* The child suddenly loses consciousness. The head slowly droops forward. If the seizure persists, the body sags forward or backward, and the patient collapses to the floor. Such attacks occur many times daily, and injuries of the head and face are common. Myoclonic seizures are also common. They may be generalized and symmetrical, as in primary generalized epilepsy, but they are also often fragmentary, characterized by twitching of the face or of one arm or leg. Generalized tonic-clonic seizures are common.

These two forms of seizures—infantile spasms and the myoclonic astatic—often disappear by the ages of eight to ten. However, tonic-clonic, myoclonic, or akinetic seizures may persist. Mental retardation occurs in 80 percent of children with this disorder, even if the seizures disappear.[9]

However, as noted above, with a subgroup showing no evidence of static or progressive encephalopathy, and without associated tonic seizures, the prognosis is more favorable, 49 percent becoming seizure-free and only 11 percent severely retarded.[10]

Adult Forms of Secondary Generalized Epilepsy. With advancing years, seizures tend to become more severe but less frequent. Generalized tonic-clonic seizures, akinetic seizures, and focal seizures are common. The general pattern continues to be one of grossly abnormal EEG and multiple seizure types with static or progressive dementia.

These difficult-to-control seizures have sometimes been spoken of as *petit mal variant.*

PROGNOSIS OF EPILEPSY

The outlook for complete control of seizures varies, depending upon the type of epilepsy, age of onset, and severity. A long-term follow-up of 457 patients[11] showed that after 15 years 61 percent had been free of seizures for five years. About 50 percent had remained seizure-free for five years without medication. Of those who had been seizure-free for five years, 2 percent relapsed each year. Thus, 90 percent of those who had been seizure-free for five years remained so for another five. The prognosis was best for those with primary generalized epilepsy, especially with onset prior to age twenty.

These studies reveal that of children with absence seizures combined with grand mal, 80 percent still "outgrow" their epilepsy. Of those with grand mal only, 85 percent become seizure-free.

For patients with complex partial (psychomotor) seizures, the prognosis is less favorable. After age twenty, 35 percent continue to have seizures. Only 35 percent have remained seizure-free for five years without medication.

The prognosis for the secondary generalized epilepsies, especially infantile spasms (West's syndrome) and the myoclonic and myoclonic astatic seizures of childhood, is especially gloomy. Over 50 to 60 percent are mentally retarded. Among children with infantile spasms, 80 percent subsequently showed IQ under 75.[12]

MORTALITY IN EPILEPSY

The reported mortality among persons with epilepsy is over two times that of the general population, and among persons with epilepsy approximately half the deaths are directly attributable to this disorder (Table 6). These figures are probably inflated, since well-controlled or arrested cases of epilepsy are often not included in such series. However, the high frequency of sudden and accidental death is noteworthy. The high suicide rate observed in many series of studies—and possibly, in fact, underreported—reflects the devastating impact of this disorder, its social repercussions, and the lack of supporting services available for this population.

THE PREVALENCE OF EPILEPSY

It is estimated that approximately 1 percent of the population has epilepsy—that is, has had at least two seizures, at least one within the past five years. Accurate figures on prevalence are difficult to obtain, since those who can tend to hide their epilepsy. Casual surveys usually uncover about four cases per thousand population. An intensive study in Rochester, Minnesota, found an overall prevalence rate of over six per thousand. It is estimated, however, that even this survey probably overlooked as many as one-third of the actual cases—those unwilling to seek medical advice or having minor

Table 6

Causes of Death of Persons with Epilepsy
Seen in Hospital Clinics and Physicians' Practices

Seizure-Related	
Accidental death—Drowning—Suicide	24%
Sudden Death Associated with Seizures	18%
Status Epilepticus	9%
Brain Disease (Tumor)	5%
Non-Neurological	41%
Unknown	3%
	100%

or nocturnal seizures of which they themselves were unaware (Table 7).[13]

Single, or sporadic seizures are much more common. From 3 to 4 percent of all children experience a febrile convulsion. By the time of death, between 5 to 8 percent of the population will have experienced at least one convulsion. This is probably an underestimate, as there are no data on the incidence of alcohol-induced seizures.

The spectrum of persons having epilepsy is a diverse one, according to age, type of epilepsy (Table 8), seizure frequency (Table 9), and associated disabilities (Table 10).

Table 7

Spectrum of Epilepsy in United States

Category	Rate/1,000	Number Affected
Total Identified with Active Epilepsy	6.6	1,409,100
Requiring ongoing medical treatment	3.6	768,600
Requiring occasional medical treatment	2.64	562,708
In residential facilities	.36	77,792
Undetected	3.4	725,900

Table 8

Relative Frequency of Various Forms of Epileptic Seizures

	Children Age 11	Adults
Petit Mal	3%	3%
Minor Only (includes Psychomotor)	20	10
Grand Mal and Others (Petit Mal)	9	11
Grand Mal and Minor (Psychomotor)	17	17
Grand Mal Only	51	59
	100	100

Table 9

Seizure Frequency in Patients with Major and Minor Seizures

Frequency	Major Seizures	Minor Seizures
One a year or less	16.3%	6.1%
Once per month to once per year	59.2%	23.5%
More than once per month	23.6	69.9%

Table 10

Associated Disabilities of Persons with Epilepsy under Active Medical Care

Epilepsy Only	23%
Mental Retardation	48%
Behavior and Adjustment Problems	54%
Neurological Deficit	10%

THE DIAGNOSIS OF EPILEPSY

Medical care for persons with epilepsy (see Table 11) starts with diagnostic evaluation. The purposes of the diagnostic evaluation are 1. to ascertain that the person has epilepsy; 2. to determine the etiology, if possible; and 3. to determine the nature of the epilepsy as a basis for therapy.

Differential Diagnosis

The following conditions must be differentiated from epilepsy:

Breath-holding Attacks in Childhood. Young children may hold their breath long enough to lose consciousness and even to have a brief anoxic seizure. Such attacks occur in response to trauma or emotional insult. Commonly the child starts crying, then holds his or her breath until unconsciousness supervenes. An actual convulsion is very rare; when present, it occurs as a brief twitching after a period of asphyxia.

Syncope. Syncopal (fainting) attacks may be quite difficult to distinguish from seizures, especially since they also may be associated with a brief convulsive phase due to cerebral asphyxia. They usually occur in young people. They are commonly triggered by pain or emotional stimulus (venipuncture, sight of blood, lacerations, or other painful injury). Pallor and profuse sweating are prominent, and recovery is immediate upon assuming the reclining position.

Heart Block. In older people, cardiac irregularities may cause episodes of cerebral ischemia most difficult to distinguish from certain seizures. Loss of consciousness may be preceded by an "aura" of dizziness, confusion, or aphasia. Such episodes occur only in older people. They do not cause unconsciousness when the patient is reclining. Definitive differentiation may require EEG or 24-hour cardiac monitor.

Transient Ischemic Attacks. Patients with cervical or cerebral arteriosclerosis experience transitory episodes of focal cerebral ischemia which may

Table 11

Medical Services—Minimum Standards of Care

Minimum standards of medical care must be adhered to for services available to any person—whether residing in an institution or in other parts of the community. These standards are outlined as follows:

I. Initial Medical Evaluation
    A. To determine the cause and nature of the epileptic process
        1. Medical history
        2. Accurate subjective and objective description of seizures
        3. Developmental history
        4. Family history
        5. Physical and neurological examination
        6. Diagnostic tests
            a. Biochemical, hematologic and serologic studies
                (1) Complete blood count
                (2) Urinalysis
                (3) Serum calcium and phosphorus
                (4) Studies to exclude tuberculosis and syphilis
                (5) Fasting blood sugar
            b. Electrophysiologic studies
                (1) Electroencephalogram (EEG)
            c. Radiologic studies
                (1) Computed tomogram of brain
                (2) Angiogram or pneumoencephalogram (if indicated)
    B. The following additional studies may be required in selected cases
        1. Five-hour glucose tolerance test for atypical seizures
        2. Chromosome studies for congenital malformations
        3. Amino acid screen for metabolic disorders
        4. Spinal fluid examination for infection of nervous system
        5. Special EEG activation procedures
            a. Sleep deprived
            b. Telemetered
            c. Chemical activation
    C. Application of International Seizure Classification
    D. Data base entry of medical problems not directly related to epileptic process

II. To Achieve Control of Seizures
    A. Reliable and accurate record of seizure frequency
    B. Charting of anticonvulsant drug consumption
    C. Periodic anticonvulsant drug levels
    D. Case review
        1. For incompletely controlled patients
            a. Weekly by technical specialist
            b. Monthly by medical specialist
        2. For patients having less than one seizure per month (for patients in

community-based living arrangements, periodic review by a physician no fewer than two times per year)
   a. Monthly by technical specialist
   b. Quarterly by medical specialist

III. To Protect Against Medical Emergency
   A. Appropriate observation by trained attendant or companion
   B. Institution of ongoing and detailed training for families, associates, attendants, or health professionals responsible for the care of patients with epilepsy
   C. Health professional availability on an emergency 24-hour basis
   D. Access to emergency hospital-type care within a time considered reasonable by the standards of care for the community. For persons in institutions, or subject to severe, prolonged, or recurrent seizures, such care should be accessible within 20 minutes

IV. Referral for Special Study
Persons with atypical or "focal onset" seizures, or having evidence of underlying neurological disease, or with uncontrolled seizures (more than one per month) should be referred for special evaluation, preferably to a center specializing in epilepsy for special services as follows.
   A. Twenty-four hour video and EEG monitoring
   B. Angiography
   C. Supervised inpatient drug control
   D. Special consideration for surgical intervention

---

resemble seizures. They may be distinguished by the predominance of inhibition rather than excitatory features of the onset, by EEG, and by presence of other evidences of arteriosclerosis. A therapeutic trial with anticonvulsant drugs may be useful. Further differentiation may require angiography.

Hypoglycemia. Hypoglycemia (low blood-sugar) is a popular but probably infrequent cause of episodes of confusion or unconsciousness. Hypoglycemic episodes occur in late morning or afternoon, starting several hours after the previous meal. Patients experience weakness, dizziness, perspiration, and mental confusion. Unlike epilepsy, the onset is gradual and the episodes are likely to persist for longer than the five or ten minutes characteristic of epilepsy. The differentiation may be aided by EEG, by a five-hour glucose tolerance test, and by modification of the episode by administration of glucose at the onset of an attack.

Hysteria. It is sometimes difficult to distinguish temporal lobe epilepsy from hysteria, especially since some patients have both. Thus, the occurrence of an attack which has all the earmarks of hysteria does not rule out epilepsy. The following criteria are helpful in making this distinction (see also Chapter 2):

Pre-existing Personality: The hysterical patient is more likely to have a history including other types of hysterical behavior—abdominal surgery for unexplained abdominal pain, headache, backache, problems with personal relations.

Precipitating Factors: The hysterical seizure is more likely to be precipitated by emotional trauma, and to occur where it will have the greatest impact on the observers. True seizures characteristically occur in a completely random fashion, influenced primarily by diurnal and sleep patterns, sleep deprivation, and the menses, or occasionally by specific sensory stimulation such as flashing lights.

Pattern of the Attack: The diversity and bizarre patterns of complex partial seizures are described above. Their manifestations may be entirely subjective. However, although they differ widely from patient to patient, within the same patient the attacks are stereotyped and repetitive, recurring repeatedly in the same format with minor variations over time and varying primarily in severity and in progression.

Retrograde Amnesia: In general, persons subject to automatic behavior retain no recollection of their behavior during the event. However, this is not absolutely universal, occasional persons remaining fully aware during their minor seizures or during the aura preceding the automatism, and a few carrying out inappropriate behavior of which they subsequently retain some recollection. Persons with hysteria usually retain some dreamlike recollection of their "attacks," and recollection can be strengthened by association or hypnosis.

Occurrence of Convulsion: The history of occurrence of generalized convulsions can confirm a diagnosis of epilepsy. Many patients suffer from minor complex partial seizures for many years before the occurrence of a generalized seizure establishes the true nature of the problem.

Electroencephalogram: In hysteria the EEG is like that in the general population. The finding of EEG abnormalities, especially during a "seizure" lends strong support to a diagnosis of epilepsy. A normal tracing, however, does not rule epilepsy out (see below).

Schizophrenia: The visual hallucinations of complex partial seizures are suggestive of schizophrenia. However, the person with epilepsy sees these visions as something imposed upon rather than part of his consciousness. He or she may say "I saw my mother just as plain and lifelike as could ever be seen," but he or she does not say, "My mother came to visit me." The patient may see "scenery passing before my eyes" and may be frightened by it, but he or she knows it is not really there. It must be recognized, however, that with this form of epilepsy there is an increased incidence of psychosis, frequently with paranoid ideation.

Etiology

The physician searches for etiology in hopes of finding a curable cause. In small children, remediable causes of seizures include lead poisoning and a few metabolic disorders such as B6 deficiency or PKU. Occasional adults suffer from low-grade meningitis, collagen vascular disease, or sarcoid. Angiomatous malformations may cause seizures starting at any age. With increasing age of onset, one thinks increasingly of tumor, although cerebrovascular disease is actually the most common cause of late-onset epilepsy.

Differentiation of Seizure Types

The differentiation of seizure types is important as a clue toward etiology and as a basis for appropriate medication. Every effort should be made to classify the patient according to one of the following four major categories:

Primary Generalized. Patients in this category may have either absence, grand mal, or both. The age of onset is from two to twenty years, most commonly four to eleven. The seizures are generalized from the onset and without aura. There are no focal or neurological signs. EEG may reveal generalized dysrhythmia, fast sharp wave episodes, or 3-4/second spike-wave.

Secondary Generalized. These epilepsies, which may occur almost from birth, are recognized by the frequency and diversity of seizure types, and by grossly abnormal EEG. They are frequently associated with significant intellectual impairment.

Partial Epilepsy with Elementary Symptomatology. The hallmark of partial epilepsy is the occurrence of a local sign or aura at the onset of the attack, asymmetry of the seizure, sometimes transitory focal paralysis or deficit in the recovery phase. The most important question to ask the patient is, "What is the first thing you feel when the seizure comes?" To the observer, the question is, "What is the first thing that you notice when he begins to have an attack?" Any premonitory sensation, or anything other than sudden loss of consciousness and generalized movement, should suggest a partial rather than generalized epilepsy.

Partial Epilepsy with Complex Symptomatology. The diverse symptomatology of partial complex seizures has been outlined above. The commonest mistake in the management of epilepsy is to confuse the minor episode of complex partial epilepsy with the "absence" of primary generalized epilepsy. Remember, "all that's small's *not* petit mal." The manifestations may be confusingly similar, but the significance and the management of the two conditions are very different. In true petit mal, the onset is abrupt and without aura. The attack is usually of brief duration—from a few seconds to one to two minutes. It is primarily an arrest of activity. Although brief automatisms may occur, they usually take the form of poorly organized fumbling movements. Recovery of consciousness is abrupt, and there is no post-ictal confusion, disorientation, or amnesia for events prior to the onset of the seizures. The complex partial seizure, on the other hand, is often—but not always—preceded by aura. The seizure is characterized by organized activity—lip-smacking and swallowing, searching movements, body spasm or torsion, or akinesis—or by various forms of complex behavior. The attack may be of only a few seconds' duration, but frequently lasts up to ten or fifteen minutes. Return of consciousness is gradual, often with a significant period of disorientation and amnesia for prior events. Differentiation may be further assisted by EEG.

Diagnostic Procedures

Essential clinical and laboratory procedures for the study of persons with epilepsy are outlined under Minimum Medical Standards (Table 11). A detailed history, a careful search for etiological factors, and a precise description of the characteristics of the seizure, especially its onset, are essential. The physical and neurological examinations are to search for underlying physical and neurological disorders relevant to etiology.

The Electroencephalogram. The electroencephalogram is the most valuable confirmatory laboratory test for epilepsy, providing valuable information regarding both the presence of epilepsy and the form or nature of the process. However, the finding of even a clearly abnormal record is not proof that the subject has overt epilepsy, and the finding of a normal EEG does not rule it out.

All degrees of abnormality may be observed in the EEG, ranging from those which are seen almost exclusively in epileptic populations and only rarely in control groups to those whose prevalence is so high in control populations as to provide little value in differentiation. Unfortunately, many electroencephalographers do not clearly distinguish these degrees of abnormality in their report. In some reports, findings are characterized as "abnormal" which are to be found in 20-40 percent of a control population. It is therefore most important for those relying on EEG interpretations to obtain a clear description of the nature of the abnormality and its degree of significance.

The following abnormalities are highly significant and lend strong support to a clinical diagnosis of epilepsy:

Generalized spike-wave discharges. The most striking and diagnostic epileptic abnormality is the paroxysmal appearance of high voltage bilaterally synchronous rhythmic 2-4/second spike and wave complexes. Brief episodes of this nature may occur without overt clinical signs, but those lasting more than ten or fifteen seconds are almost always associated with demonstrable impairment of consciousness. Thus, this finding is most commonly associated with primary generalized epilepsy and is almost diagnostic of an epileptic trait. However, in their studies of the inheritance of centrencephalic (primary generalized) epilepsy, Metrakos and Metrakos observed that 37 percent of the siblings of such patients had this type of EEG abnormality, while only 13 percent were known to have overt seizures. Among the siblings of a matched control population, 9 percent had the EEG trait, while only 5 percent were known to have seizures.[14] Thus, even in the presence of this striking abnormality, there are some children who are not recognized as epileptic (see Table 12).

Multiple spike-wave complexes. Multiple spike-wave and irregular spike-wave complexes carry an almost equivalent significance. Whereas the rhythmic 2-4/second discharge is most commonly associated with simple absence attacks, with or without associated tonic-clonic seizures, the multiple spike-wave pattern is more often associated with myoclonic or

Table 12

Abnormalities of EEG of Relatives of Children with "Centrencephalic" Epilepsy and of Control (Presumably "Normal") Children*

| | *Percent Affected* | | | |
| | *Parents* | | *Siblings* | |
Type of EEG	*Cases*	*Controls*	*Cases*	*Controls*
Normal	72	79	30	46
Borderline Normal	15	7	17	26
Typical Centrencephalic	1	0	2	0
Theta Rhythms	0	0	2	2
Multiple Diffuse	3	5	8	11
Focal	3	6	4	5
Others	.5	1.0	2	2
Normal and Borderline	87	86	47	72
Total Abnormal	13	14	53	28
Total Centrencephalic	7	2	37	9
Total Epileptiform	9	6	46	16
With Convulsions	14	1	13	5

*These figures include persons having febrile convulsions.

akinetic attacks. Irregular 2/second spike-waves seen in a diffusely slow record are associated with the secondary generalized epilepsies and also carry a high diagnostic significance. However, low voltage spike-wave discharges at higher frequencies—6/second and above—are seen very frequently in normal populations and carry much less diagnostic significance of epilepsy, even though they are looked upon as being epilepsy-related.

Random spike discharges. The hallmark of the partial (focal) epilepsies is the presence of random spike and wave or slow wave discharges localized to some area of the scalp. Their significance varies depending upon their voltage and the frequency of their occurrence. They may sometimes be confused with artifact or with sudden transients occurring normally at the onset of sleep. However, the presence of well-formed spikes or spike-wave discharges is a highly significant diagnostic finding.

Changes in EEG during clinical seizures. The onset of a clinical seizure is commonly associated with some change is the EEG. In patients with primary generalized epilepsy (especially absence), the attack is associated with 2-4/second spike-wave discharges. If a generalized seizure occurs in such patients, this discharge may lead to a multiple spike and generalized discharge. In other instances, tonic-clonic seizures may begin with a burst of low-voltage, fast, sharp waves or spikes. In patients with partial epilepsy, the aura may be associated with a silent period, or a sudden "flattening" of the record, followed by a crescendo burst of repetitive high frequency discharges of increasing voltage and diminishing frequency. Whatever the nature of the onset, the occurrence of a clinical seizure is ordinarily associated with a concomitant sudden change in the pattern of the EEG. Sometimes such abnormal discharges are obscured by muscle artifact. The occurrence of such changes is especially valuable in differentiating epileptic from hysterical seizures. Even here, however, there are reported instances in which a true epileptic seizure (complex parital) was associated with a subcortical electrical discharge which did not show up on scalp EEG.

The following abnormalities are seen more often in an epileptic population than among controls but, unless of marked degree, are of limited differential value because they are frequent also among the normal population.

Generalized slowing, diffuse random 3-4/second waves. The most common "dominant frequency" of the EEG is the Alpha rhythm ranging from 8-12/second. Some people have a slower or faster dominant rhythm, and slow or fast rhythms are more common in epilepsy than among controls.

Varying amounts of slow wave activity, 3-4/second random waves, are observed in most records. They are more prominent in the records of persons with epilepsy. However, such non-specific abnormalities may be engendered by drowsiness, use of drugs, or metabolic changes, including moderate hypoglycemia. In addition, they are seen in up to 20-30 percent of normal populations, depending upon the criteria of the electroenceph-alographer. Even in the careful studies of Metrakos and Metrakos (Table 12) and Metrakos,[15] it is noted that 14 percent of adults and 28 percent of children of a control population were considered to have an "abnormal" record. Six percent of adults and 16 percent of children were considered "epileptiform." Thus, except in the presence of the clear-cut epileptic discharges described above, the report of an "abnormal" EEG must be interpreted with caution if not outright skepticism.

A single normal EEG cannot be said to rule out epilepsy. In one large series of well studied patients finally diagnosed as epileptic, an abnormal record was found on the first EEG in only 40 percent.[16] With repeated tracings, especially those associated with sleep or sleep-deprivation, the percentage may reach 60 percent. Even higher figures may be achieved with hospitalization, withdrawal of medication, and 24-hour monitoring. Abnormal EEG is found more commonly in children with epilepsy than in epileptic adults; however, these data reveal that in the adult with known epilepsy it is more likely than not that the record will be normal.

The CAT X-ray Scan. Another laboratory test whose importance cannot be overestimated in the CAT x-ray scan. Within one large series of epileptic patients, 50 percent exhibited abnormalities of this scan—8 to 11 percent had tumors.[17] Table 13 shows these data. The Commission for the Control of Epilepsy and Its Consequences has recommended that every person with epilepsy have the benefit of this evaluation to make certain that no tumor or other remedial cause of epilepsy be overlooked.

The power of the CAT x-ray scan is so great that radioisotope scans now

Table 13

Frequencies of Cerebral Lesions Demonstrated
by CAT in 401 Patients with Epilepsy

Type Epilepsy	% with Cerebral Lesion
Partial	63
Grand Mal (Primary and Secondary)	43
Primary Generalized (Absence)	10
All Grouped	50

have little additional to contribute—although new techniques using positron-emission for the study of localized changes in metabolic rate offer promise of great value in determining the site of a focal epileptic discharge. Pneumoencephalogram and angiogram are primarily preoperative procedures, or used where there is strong evidence of vascular malformation or tumor.[18]

TREATMENT OF SEIZURES: ANTICONVULSANT DRUGS

The most important measure for the control of epileptic seizures is the use of anticonvulsant drugs. The objective is to achieve complete seizure control with minimum side effects. The specific drugs required and their dosage vary with the nature of the epilepsy and the individual. For this reason, there are no hard and fast rules for drug selection or dosage; a considerable period of drug manipulation may be required before the best drug or drug combination is achieved. There are, however, certain principles that should be observed.

Starting Medication

Once a person is started on anticonvulsant drugs, he or she is committed to continue medication for a minimum of three to four years. For this reason, medication should not be started until the diagnosis of recurrent seizures has been established. There is controversy as to whether a patient should be started on medication after a single seizure.

Follow-up studies revealed that among a group of individuals who experienced a single "spontaneous" epileptic seizure, 25 percent experienced a second attack during the ensuing two years, and one-third within thirty months. The presence of abnormality of EEG was found to be a poor predictor of recurrences. However, the recurrences occurred earlier in those patients with "symptomatic" seizures and with a positive family history.[19]

Findings in children are similar.[20] Among a group of 71 children whose first seizure occurred from birth to age sixteen, only 28 (39 percent) had no second seizure; 19 (27 percent) had had a seizure within the year preceding the follow-up (see Table 14).

Data from the "kindling" experiments suggest that repeated seizures predispose to more seizures, and that this progressive lowering of seizure threshold can be prevented by appropriate anticonvulsant drugs.[21] For this reason, where there is an abnormal EEG following a single seizure, or at the earliest time when a diagnosis can be established, medication should be started. Special urgency relates to infantile spasms. Immediate treatment appears critical in hopes of arresting the malignant course of this disorder.

Table 14

Three-year Follow-up after Single Seizure in Children*

	Number	Percent
Frequency of Recurrence		
Single Seizure Only	28	39
Recurrent Seizures	43	61
Total	71	100
Seizure Control Among Those Whose Seizures Recurred		
Seizure-free One Year without Medication	3	4
Seizure-free One Year with Medication	21	30
Recurrent Seizures within the Previous Year	19	27
Total with Recurrent Seizures	43	61

Starting and Stopping

For most drugs, side effects are minimized if the dosage is built up gradually. It is wise to start with a single drug and increase that drug to tolerance level, adding additional medication if control is not achieved, or gradually substituting if the initial drug proves ineffectual. Except in the case of life-threatening drug sensitivity, *an anticonvulsant drug should never be terminated abruptly.* To do so offers the risk of precipitating status epilepticus—a condition of repeated or continuous seizures carrying mortality up to 40 percent in some series.[22] If a drug is to be discontinued, it should be reduced gradually over a period of weeks or months.

Compliance

The commonest cause of status epilepticus is failure of compliance. After a seizure-free period, the ill-advised patient convinces him or herself that he or she doesn't need medicine; or the patient runs out of medicine and doesn't realize its importance. Studies show that as many as 30 percent of treated patients are not following instructions.[23] For these reasons, it is absolutely essential that at the time drug therapy is initiated, and repeatedly thereafter, the physician discuss frankly and in detail with the patient the need for drug treatment, the necessity of maintaining an adequate drug level, that the aim is control and not cure, and that continued medication will be required for a period of years after complete control is achieved.

The use of blood level determinations of anticonvulsant drugs provides a valuable monitor of drug compliance, and such measures should be used whenever there is unexpected recurrence of seizures, as well as at the time when effective seizure control is achieved or during the regulation of drug dosage. Again, the commonest cause of inappropriate drug levels is noncompliance. However, it should not be overlooked that unusual idiosyncrasies of drug absorption or drug interactions may also produce unexpectedly high or low levels, and a patient should not be treated for noncompliance until these other factors have been carefully assessed.

Toxic Side Effects

Few drugs can be given in large doses and for long periods of time without the possibility of toxic side effects. In the case of patients on anticonvulsant drugs, both the physician and the patient should be aware of the potential side effects of the drugs. The patient should be advised that in the event of any intercurrent illness, the possibility of toxic drug effect should be considered and a physician knowledgeable about the patient's medication should be consulted. Physicians prescribing for other illnesses should always have brought to their attention the possibility of drug interactions in persons with epilepsy. This problem also applies in respect to the use of psychotropic drugs, some of which interfere with the excretion of anticonvulsant drugs, causing them to build up to toxic levels.

Commonly recognized interactions among various anticonvulsant drugs are listed in Table 15 and interactions of phenytoin (Dilantin) with other types of drugs in Table 16. Probably the most striking effect is the enhancement of phenytoin level which occurs following the administration of isoniazid for the treatment of tuberculosis in persons already under treatment for epilepsy. The sudden rise in phenytoin level which occurs when isoniazid is added may produce severe toxic effects which if unrecognized have resulted in irreversible cerebellar damage.

The interactions of anticonvulsant drugs with tranquillizers are rather unpredictable and less dramatic. Phenothiazines may produce some lowering in seizure threshold, often accompanied by a slight lowering of anticonvulsant drug levels. (Haloperidol is reported to cause some increase in levels.) For this reason, it is wise to monitor drug levels when a tranquillizer is added, and to adjust the dosage levels of the anticonvulsant accordingly. In general, the fact that an epileptic person is receiving anticonvulsant drugs is no contraindication to the use of tranquillizers.

Table 15

Summary of Potential Interactions Between One Antiepileptic Drug and Another

Drug Affected	Interfering Drug	Probable Mechanism	Potential Result
Interactions increasing antiepileptic drug levels			
Phenytoin Phenobarbitone Primidone	Sulthiame	Inhibition of metabolism	Rise in serum level of affected drug—producing enhanced therapeutic effect at a risk of causing drug intoxication
Phenytoin Phenobarbitone	Pheneturide	Inhibition of metabolism	
Phenobarbitone Primidone	Sodium Valproate	Inhibition of metabolism	30% rise in phenobarbitone level
Phenytoin	Sodium Valproate	Displacement from plasma protein binding sites	Rise in free (not total) level of affected drug—producing transient increase in drug effects
Phenytoin Phenobarbitone	Phenobarbitone Phenytoin	Inhibition or stimulation of metabolism	Variable
Interactions decreasing antiepileptic drug levels			
Phenytoin	Carbamazepine	Induction of metabolism of affected drug	Reduced serum level of affected drug usually not of clinical importance because of added effect of interfering drug
Phenytoin	Diazepam Clonazepam		
Diazepam Clonazepam Carbamazepine Sodium Valproate	Phenytoin Phenobarbitone Primidone Carbamazepine Pheneturide		
Primidone	Phenytoin	Induction of metabolism	Conversion to phenobarbitone stimulated

Table 16

Drugs that Have Been Observed to Elevate DPH Plasma Levels

Other drug Name	Dose mg/day	No. of patients	DPH dose per day	DPH level (µg/ml) before giving other drug Range	Average	DPH level (µg/ml) during administration of other drug Range	Average
Bishydroxycoumarin	to give prothrombine value of 30%	1	300 mg	—	21	—	40
"	400-800	5	300 mg	4-7	5.3	12-17	15.1
Phenyramidol	1200	5	300 mg	4-10	7	8-14	12.1
Disulfiram	400-800	3	300-400 mg	11-20	15	33-51	39
"	400	4	300-400 mg	4-16	7.2	18-36	25
"	400	2	300-350 mg	18-20	19	27-29	28
Sulthiame	200-800	4	300 mg	7-12	10	17-28	22
"	400-600	7	unknown	4-14	9	8-24	18
Chloramphenicol	2000	2	250 mg	2-3	2.5	7-11	9
Methylphenidate	20-40	1	8.9 mg/kg	—	9	—	28
Chlordiazepoxide or diazepam	unknown	1	300-400 mg	—	19.8	—	41.2
"	unknown	4	300-400 mg	4-14	10	11-20	16
Isoniazid	300	34	300 mg	8-20	12	34-61	42

Specific Drugs Used in the Treatment of Epilepsy

Table 17 depicts the dosage forms of commonly used anticonvulsant drugs, the dosage range, desirable drug levels, and evidences of toxicity. Following are the drug characteristics and uses:

√ *Barbiturates: Phenobarbital, Primidone (Mysoline), Metharbital (Mebaral).* The barbiturates have the advantage of a broad spectrum of effectiveness, prolonged action, and rare sensitization. They are commonly used for both primary and secondary generalized (tonic-clonic) seizures and for the partial epilepsies. They are not helpful in absence seizures. Primidone and metharbital are converted to penobarbital in the body and are thus similar to but not identical with phenobarbital in their action. Primidone is especially effective for complex partial seizures, although its effects are primarily those of phenobarbital.

The major drawback with the barbiturates is their sedative effect. In adults this produces dullness of intellect, depression, and drowsiness; in children, hyperactivity, aggressiveness, and irritability. Barbiturates also occasionally produce dermatitis and acne. All these effects can be intolerable. In addition, animal experiments have demonstrated impaired brain growth in infant rats receiving therapeutic doses of phenobarbital. For these reasons, many physicians try to avoid the barbiturates when possible.

√ *Hydantoins: Phenytoin (Dilantin), Mephenytoin (Mesantoin), Ethotoin (Peganone).* Phenytoin is effective against all forms of tonic-clonic seizures, and especially effective in preventing the spread of partial seizures, both elementary and complex. It is far less sedative than phenobarbital. In overdosage it produces a cerebellar form of ataxia—there is unsteadiness of eye movement (nystagmus) and a drunken gait. Overdosage may be accompanied by paradoxical enhancement of seizures, and unless monitored by drug level determinations, the temptation to try to control seizures by further increasing the dosage may lead to an ever-worsening situation. Reduction in dosage may actually improve seizure control. There is some suggestion that severe overdosage may lead to irreversible cerebellar damage.[24]

Phenytoin regularly produces gum hypertrophy and hirsutism—the latter particularly disturbing to women. Mephenytoin does not share these effects; however, it occasionally produces dangerous blood leukopenia, and its use is thus reserved for patients with intolerable gum hypertrophy or uncontrollable complex partial seizures, for some of whom it may be superior to phenytoin.

When given to children over long periods of time, phenytoin produces characteristic facial deformities—protruding teeth, thick lips, and flattened nose and forehead,[25] and this syndrome has also recently been discovered in infants of women taking phenytoin during pregnancy (see page 40). In adults, prolonged medication may also produce a mild peripheral neuropathy, further increasing the ataxia. Prolonged phenytoin administration may also be associated with increased frequency of lymphoma.[26] Sensitivity to phenytoin is also common and may lead to severe dermatitis, the Stevens-Johnson syndrome, or lupus erythematosus. Agranulocytosis also occurs. The occurrence of any of these is an indication for immediate withdrawal of the drug.

Succinimides: Ethosuximide (Zarontin), Methsuximide (Celontin), Phensuximide (Milontin). These drugs are all well tolerated. In large doses they produce drowsiness or ataxia. Ethosuximide is the drug of choice for absence seizures, especially since it also contributes to the control of tonic-clonic (grand mal) seizures of primary generalized epilepsy. Methsuximide is useful in myoclonic seizures and complex partial seizures. Sensitivity is rare. Overdosage may be associated also with headache, muscle pains, or generalized weakness.

Carbamazepine (Tegretol). Carbamazepine, a close relative of imipramine, is finding increasing usefulness in the control of tonic-clonic seizures as well as various forms of partial epilepsy. It is also occasionally effective for unusual absence seizures but is not commonly prescribed for this type of epilepsy. Thus its effectiveness is comparable to that of phenytoin, which it is increasingly supplanting. In overdoses, it produces double vision and dizziness. Sensitization, manifested by dermatitis or aphthous ulcers of the mouth, is common. Moderate depression of the bone marrow with lowered white count is very common, but unless the WBC falls below 3,000 is not an indication for discontinuation of the drug. Agranulocytosis and hepatitis have been reported, and for this reason repeated blood counts are recommended. This drug is useful because it does not have the sedative effects of phenobarbital or cause the changes of appearance seen with phenytoin. In Europe it is considered by many the drug of choice for certain forms of childhood epilepsy, but there are as yet not sufficient studies in children in the USA to support its approval for such use by the FDA.

Diones: Trimethadione (Tridione), Paramethadione (Paradione). Until the development of ethosuximide, the diones were the only drugs available specifically for the treatment of absence seizures. They are now drugs of last resort for that type of epilepsy, although there may be rare instances where individuals resistant to ethosuximide or valproic acid may respond

Table 17
Anticonvulsant Drugs

NAME	AVERAGE ADULT DAILY DOSE	FORM	SIDE EFFECTS	TYPE OF SEIZURE BENEFITED			
				Major Motor	Minor Motor	Petit Mal	Psychomotor
ATABRINE	100 mg.	50-100 mg./tablet	Yellow discoloration of skin; diarrhea, nausea	-	-	+	-
CELONTIN	300 mg. - 1.2 gm.	150-300 mg. Kapseals	Blood dyscrasias, nausea, anorexia, ataxia, rash, drowsiness, dizziness	-	-	+	-
CLONOPIN	1.5-20 mg.	0.5-1-2 mg. tablets	Drowsiness, ataxia, behavior changes, tremor, depression, hair loss, hirsutism, anorexia	-	+	+	-
DEPAKENE	1750-3000 mg.	250 mg. Kapseal	Gastro-intestinal disturbance, altered bleeding time, liver toxicity	+	+	+	-
DESOXYN	5-10 mg.	5-10-15 mg. Gradumet Tablets 2.5-5 mg. tablet	Anorexia, irritability, insomnia, tachycardia, tremor, headache	+	-	+	+
DEXEDRINE	5-15 mg.	5-10-15 mg. 'spansule' capsules 5-10-15 mg. tablets	Anorexia, irritability, insomnia, tachycardia, tremor, headache	+	-	+	+
DIAMOX	250-1000 mg.	125-250-1000 mg. tablets 500 mg. Sequels	Numbness of extremities, anorexia, polyuria, drowsiness, confusion	+	-	+	-

Drug	Daily Dose	Preparation	Side Effects				
DILANTIN	100-400 mg.	30-100 mg. Kapseal / 30-125 mg. Suspension / 50 mg. Infatabs 100 mg. Dilantin c/¼ or ½ gr. Phenobarbital Kapseals	Ataxia, insomnia, motor twitching, nausea, rash, gingival hyperplasia, hirsutism	+	+	-	+
GEMONIL	100-800 mg.	100 mg. tablets	Gastric distress, dizziness, irritability, rash, drowsiness	+	+	+	+
LIBRIUM	30-75 mg.	5-10-25 mg. capsule	Drowsiness, ataxia, rash, edema, nausea	+	+	+	+
MEBARAL	400-600 mg.	32-50-100-200 mg. tablet	Dizziness, headache, nausea, facial edema, skin rash	+	-	+	-
MESANTOIN	0.2-0.6 Gm.	100 mg. tablet	Blood dyscrasias, skin rashes, ataxia, diplopia, tremor, drowsiness	+	-	-	+
MYSOLINE	250-1000 mg.	50-250 mg. tablet 250 mg. suspension per 5 cc	Ataxia, vertigo, anorexia, fatigue, drowsiness, hyperirritability	+	-	-	+
PARADIONE	600 mg.-2.4 Gm.	150-300 mg. capsules	Nausea, anorexia, insomnia, diplopia, skin rash, bleeding gums, blood dyscrasias	-	-	+	-
PEGANONE	2-3 Gm.	250-500 mg. tablets	Nausea, fatigue, insomnia, diplopia, skin rash, fever, headache, dizziness, numbness	+	+	-	+
PHENOBARBITAL	100 mg.	15-30-60-100 mg. tablet	Drowsiness, irritability	+	+	+	+

Table 17 (continued)

Drug	Dose	Form	Side Effects				
PHENURONE	2-3 Gm.	500 mg. tablet	Anorexia, drowsiness, insomnia, psychic changes, hepatitis, nephritis, blood dyscrasias	+	+	+	+
RITALIN	20-30 mg.	5-10-20 mg. tablet	Nervousness, insomnia, skin rash, nausea, dizziness, abdominal pain, headache	+	-	+	+
TEGRETOL	600-1200 mg.	200 mg. tablet	Dizziness, drowsiness, blurred vision, nausea, anorexia, skin rashes, blood dyscrasias	+	-	-	+
TRANXENE	15-45 mg.	3.75-7.50-15 mg. capsules SD 11.25 mg. - SD 22.50 mg.	Drowsiness, fatigue, ataxia, depression, headache, tremor	+	+	+	+
TRIDIONE	600 mg., 2-4Gm.	300 mg. capsule 150 mg. dulcet (chewable)	Nausea, anorexia, insomnia, diplopia, skin rash, bleeding gums, blood dyscrasias	-	-	+	-
VALIUM	4-40 mg.	2-5-10 mg. tablet	Drowsiness, fatigue, ataxia, depression, headache, tremor	+	+	+	+
ZARONTIN	500 mg., 1.5 Gm.	250 mg. capsule syrup 250 mg. per 5 cc	Anorexia, nausea, drowsiness, headache, dizziness, fatigue,	-	-	+	-

to trimethadione or paramethadione. The major problem with the diones is the occasional occurrence of fatal agranulocytosis due to bone marrow sensitization. In addition, it has been recently reported that over 80 percent of children born to women taking trimethadione suffered from significant congenital malformation. Its use is now rarely indicated.

Benzodiazepines: Diazepam (Valium), Clonazepam (Clonopin). Diazepam is a powerful anticonvulsant drug, especially effective when given parenterally to control status epilepticus. Its major side effect is lethargy, especially in the initial doses. Toxic or sensitivity reactions are very rare.

Clonazepam is a closely related drug, even more powerful than diazepam and with similar side effects. It produces, in addition, increased salivation and bronchial secretion.

These drugs have usefulness as adjunctive treatment in the absence seizures of primary generalized epilepsy, in the secondary generalized epilepsies (especially infantile spasms), and for the control of myoclonic and occasionally complex partial seizures. Unfortunately, although their initial effects may be dramatic, tolerance frequently develops, and their beneficial effects may be lost. Aggressive and irritable behavior is common, sometimes to the point of requiring discontinuation of the drug. Sudden withdrawal of diazepam or clonazepam may lead to a condition of "petit mal status"—the state of continued absence attacks appearing as mental confusion.

Valproic Acid (Depakene). Valproic acid is a new addition to the U.S. Pharmacopeia, and its effectiveness and long-range toxicity have not yet been fully assessed, although it has been in use in France and other countries since 1965. It is most effective in the primary generalized epilepsies, has some value in the secondary generalized epilepsies, and may be helpful as adjunctive treatment in the partial epilepsies. Thus, it has an extremely broad range of usefulness. Overdosage may produce somnolence and a Parkinson-like tremor. The commonest side effects are nausea and vomiting, temporary loss of hair, and obesity. Diminution of platelet count is common, but excessive bleeding has not been reported. The greatest concern relates to hepatic effects; lowered fibrinogen levels are almost universal, and fatal cases of hepatitis have been reported.[27] For this reason, repeated liver function tests are desirable, and patients should be on the alert for aggravation of gastrointestinal complaints and jaundice.

In spite of these uncommon side effects, valproic acid is well tolerated by most patients. In therapeutic doses it has little sedative effect. When it can be used to replace phenobarbital, there may result a dramatic lifting of somnolence and depression. Its results in resistant absence and myoclonic seizures may be impressive.

When valproic acid is added to the existing medication with pheno-barbital or primidone, there is a drug interaction leading to increased phenobarbital levels usually amounting to about 30 percent. For this reason, as the valproic dosage is gradually increased, phenobarbital must be reduced. Otherwise the patient may experience increased somnolence which can easily be falsely attributed to the newly added valproic acid.

Phenacemide (Phenurone). Phenacemide is a powerful anticonvulsant drug, especially effective against complex partial seizures. However, its use-fulness is sharply limited because of common and serious side effects. Patients receiving phenacemide frequently develop psychotic behavior with paranoia and hallucinosis. The process is reversible with withdrawal of the drug. Hepatitis is also not uncommon. For these reasons phen-acemide has limited usefulness. However, for occasional patients with complex partial seizures it may be the only effective medication.

Drug Use during Pregnancy

The risk of congenital defect is significantly increased in the children of women taking anticonvulsant drugs. The risk takes two forms. Trimetha-dione, phenytoin, and phenobarbital carry an increased risk of major con-genital malformation such as cleft palate and congenital heart disease. Phenytoin and phenobarbital also produce the "fetal hydantoin syndrome" consisting of coarseness of features and maldevelopment of fingernails. These abnormalities have been reported in frequencies ranging up to 40 percent in some series. In one series there was also reported a ten-point lowering in IQ in children whose mothers were taking anticonvulsant drugs as com-pared to their siblings born without exposure to these medications (see Table 18).

Trimethadione appears to produce an extremely high frequency of mal-formation (up to 80 percent), and in view of the availability of other more effective drugs for absence seizures, its use in women of childbearing age no longer seems justifiable. Adequate data are not yet available regarding possible teratogenetic effects of the less widely used drugs and of carba-mazepine and valproic acid. However, both of these latter drugs have been shown to be teratogenic in animals.

Drug Therapy In Epileptic Psychoses—Summary (See also Chapters 3 and 4)

It is important to distinguish three different forms of epileptic psychosis, namely the ictal, the post-ictal and the inter-ictal.

Table 18

Incidence of Drug-induced Malformations

Reference	# Studied	% Malformation	% Stigmata	
Hanson et al., 1976	35	11	31	
Visser et al., 1976				
Prior to 1945	54	4		
1959-1968	65	15		
			Digital hypoplasia	Dermal arch.
Dansky et al., 1977				
Off medicine		6.5	9	2.1
On medicine		15.2	22	18.7
Biale et al., 1975	56	16		
Koppe et al., 1973	197	13		

Ictal Forms. During their seizures, the automatic behavior of persons with complex partial seizures (psychomotor) is sometimes mistakenly looked upon as psychotic behavior. The seizure is easily recognized by its sudden, spontaneous, unprovoked onset, and brief duration—ordinarily under 15 minutes. The patient is subsequently amnestic for the events. Behavior is unplanned and inappropriate. Aggressive goal-directed activities are extremely rare.

Demented behavior may occur in association with *epilepsia partialis continua* or partial status epilepticus. There are two forms—those with continuous absence seizures (absence status), and those with continuous complex partial seizures (psychomotor status). These episodes are associated with confusion and clouded consciousness. Diagnosis can be established by EEG.

The treatment for the ictal forms of psychosis is the control of seizures by appropriate anticonvulsant medication. Partial status epilepticus ordinarily responds dramatically to intravenous diazepam—the response being sufficiently specific to provide a further verification of the diagnosis.

Post-ictal Forms. Many patients are confused and disoriented in the post-ictal period, and may remain so for rather prolonged periods of time. In fact there are reported instances (termed poriomania) in which patients have traveled for days or weeks with subsequent amnesia for the entire period. It is believed that these amnestic episodes are preceded by a seizure—sometimes subclinical.

Patients may be aggressive if accosted during a post-ictal confusional state.

Post-ictal psychosis are ordinarily self-limited, and do not require medication. They are best prevented by use of the appropriate anticonvulsant medication for the control of the underlying seizure disorder.

Inter-ictal Psychosis. One of the most serious complications of epilepsy is the development of the late-onset paranoid-hallucinatory psychosis. Unlike the previously outlined confusional states, this condition is a true psychosis and may occur in patients who are not demented, confused, or amnestic. The condition is often associated with considerable insight. Furthermore, although patients show many features suggestive of schizophrenia, the basic personality is not schizoid—there is appropriate affect. The basic characteristics of this psychosis are outlined in Table 19.

A remarkable feature of this phenomenon is that it sometimes bears reciprocal relationship with seizure frequency. The psychosis becomes worse when the seizures are controlled (and the EEG is more normal—a process called "forced normalization"). The recurrence of seizures may be associated with disappearance of the psychosis. Thus, in this condition the problem is more likely to result from *too much* medication rather than too little. It is best treated by reduction of depressant drugs such as primidone or phenobarbital and even the hydantoins, and by substitution of carbamezapine (Tegretol) or sometimes valproic acid (Depakene). In addition, there are suggestions that a dopaminergic mechanism may be involved and these psychoses respond very favorably to antipsychotic drugs such as haloperidol (Haldol) or thioridazine (Mellaril).

The other common form of inter-ictal psychosis is that due to drug intox-

Table 19

Paranoid-Hallucinatory Psychoses

Onset 0-44 years (Median 18) after onset of epilepsy
Sometimes resemble the aura of complex partial seizures
Spike focus in medial-basal temporal region—often bilateral
Increased slow wave in waking EEG record
Often periodic—may be associated with improvement of EEG
    ("forced normalization")
Reciprocal relationship with seizure frequency
Respond to antipsychotic agents

ication. Overdose with barbiturates or phenytoin may cause extreme leth-argy, confusion and ataxia. Its true nature may be overlooked when sudden increases in anticonvulsant drug levels occur as a result of administration of other medication—especially isoniazide. The condition may be diagnosed by measurement of anticonvulsant drug levels, and treated by proper drug regulation.

OTHER TREATMENT METHODS: SURGERY

In properly selected cases, surgical removal of that part of the brain con-taining an epileptic focus can provide relief in 60 to 70 percent of cases.[28] The indications for surgery are:

1. Partial epilepsy.
2. Focus located in a site accessible to surgical removal.
3. Seizures uncontrolled after thorough trial of drug therapy.

The detection of the primary focus is a specialized and difficult undertaking which may require 24-hour monitoring with or without implantation of depth electrodes. Patients should be referred to centers specializing in these pro-cedures if surgery is contemplated. Best results have been obtained with patients exhibiting a single type of seizure and those whose epilepsy is of short duration. For this reason, early operation is being increasingly rec-ommended.[29]

OTHER TREATMENT METHODS: HEALTH HABITS

Sleep deprivation is a precipitating cause of seizures in some patients. Regularity of sleep should be encouraged. Large amounts of alcohol can produce seizures, and the hydrating effects of beer are undesirable. Small amounts of alcohol are tolerated by some patients.

OTHER TREATMENT METHODS: "PSYCHOLOGICAL"

The relation between emotional factors and seizures and the treatment of epilepsy by "psychological" means are discussed in Chapter 2.

TREATMENT OF FEBRILE CONVULSIONS

One of the commonest forms of epileptic seizures is that occurring in association with febrile illnesses of childhood. From 3 to 5 percent of all children have a febrile seizure. Fortunately, the occurrence of a single seizure does little if any harm.[30] However, in instances of pre-existing brain damage, the febrile convulsion may be followed by neurological deficit or recurrent epilepsy. For this reason, children who have experienced a febrile seizure and who are considered likely to suffer damage from subsequent attacks may be treated with prophylactic anticonvulsants. In this particular instance, phenytoin is of no value. Phenobarbital, in doses sufficient to maintain a blood level above 15 mcg./ml. is effective in preventing subsequent febrile attacks.[31] It is ordinarily continued until the age of 5, following which the risk of recurrent febrile attacks ceases. It is tempting to consider giving phenobarbital only at the time of the recurrent febrile illness. However, experience has demonstrated that phenobarbital is too slowly absorbed to be effective if given at the onset of a recognized febrile illness. Diazepam as rectal suppository is a more rapidly acting drug which can be given prophylactically at the onset of a febrile illness.[32]

Management of a Febrile Convulsion

Ordinarily, a febrile convulsion is a self-limited episode consisting of a generalized tonic-clonic seizure of under five minutes duration. Seizures which are unilateral in character or of longer duration are suggestive of underlying brain damage and carry a more serious prognosis. The persistence of an attack beyond five to ten minutes constitutes a medical emergency which demands prompt intervention and immediate seizure control by the use of intravenous diazepam or phenobarbital. In any instance of febrile convulsion where question exists regarding the nature of the febrile illness, lumbar puncture or other appropriate studies are required to be certain that the convulsion is not the result of brain disease rather than a non-specific response to fever.

EMERGENCY TREATMENT OF SEIZURES

One of the most disturbing features of some convulsions is the sense of helplessness that they engender in those who observe them. As a result, people may do too much rather than too little to help.

Grand Mal Seizures

The ordinary grand mal convulsion is a self-limited episode lasting five to ten minutes and without serious sequelae. Persons having a convulsion should be slid away from hard or dangerous abjects, and the head should be protected from the floor or other rough surfaces by padded clothing or other soft objects. If possible, the body and head should be turned to one side to encourage drainage of saliva and vomitus from the airway. As the subject relaxes and breathing commences, the jaw may be drawn forward by pressure from behind the mandible just below the ears.

Tongue-biting is a disturbing feature of some attacks. Patients who have an aura may sometimes protect themselves against this by biting down on a soft object like a handkerchief *before* the actual attack starts. Once the patient has become rigid in the attack, efforts to force objects into the mouth are only damaging to the teeth. It is best to keep your hands away from the patient's mouth. You can only do harm.

After the attack, most patients are confused, disoriented, and sleepy. They should be stimulated as little as possible and permitted to sleep it off if they will, or to go about their regular activities if they prefer. A common mistake is to call an ambulance and coerce the patient into it. The confused person not infrequently becomes belligerent if manhandled during the recovery phase of a seizure.

Complex Partial Seizures

Complex partial (psychomotor) seizures with automatism commonly start with arrest of movement or repetitive movements of the face or hands lasting one to two minutes. Automatic semipurposeful activities may ensue and persist for five to ten minutes. During this period, the subject may wander aimlessly, fumble with clothing or objects in the environment, or even start running (running fits). If these actions are blocked, or especially if efforts are made to restrain or coerce the subject, he or she may become disturbed and even violent. For this reason, except in life-threatening situations the patient should be permitted to move about unrestrained until the attack is over. As the patient regains contact with the environment, he or she may be reassured with quiet words and matter-of-fact discussion and reorientation.

Persistent Seizures: Status Epilepticus

Seizures which persist for over ten to fifteen minutes, or which recur without intervening restoration of consciousness, carry the threat of status epilepticus and require prompt intervention. For some patients this is a characteristic pattern—a single seizure heralding a series of attacks which may last all day. For such subjects, the use of oral or intramuscular diazepam administered after the initial attack can interrupt the cycle and limit the process to a single seizure.

When a seizure lasts for more than ten or fifteen minutes, it should be arrested by intravenous medication. If facilities for such are not available, intramuscular diazepam is a more dangerous and less prompt alternative which can be administered prior to transportation to hospital or emergency clinic. Under no circumstances should seizures be permitted to continue beyond this period without active intervention.

EPILEPSY AND INHERITANCE

In 1978 a New York court decided that a physician who fails to advise his or her patient of the possible risk of an unfavorable outcome of pregnancy has financial responsibility for the lifetime care of a handicapped child. The courts have thus documented what should long have been considered a professional and moral responsibility of physicians.

The limits of this responsibility still remain to be defined, especially where the degree of genetic risk involved is uncertain. It is clear that the physician owes it to the patient to make available current knowledge regarding genetic risks relative to any disorder in which such factors may play a significant role. Epilepsy is such a condition.

But counseling for epilepsy is a very difficult undertaking, primarily because epilepsy is a symptom of many different disorders, and the genetic risk depends upon the nature of the underlying disease.[33] In addition, it is not the seizure itself which may be inherited but, if anything, a susceptibility to seizures. Some forms of epilepsy occur in persons subject to a well-defined inherited disease. Even in such cases the expression of epilepsy varies according to unpredictable additional genetic and environmental factors. In the majority of cases of epilepsy we are not dealing with a clear-cut "single gene" phenomenon. There appear to be within the population all degrees of constitutionally determined susceptibility to seizures. The occurrence of seizures within a given individual depends upon the interaction of his or her constitution with a complex of environmental factors, including physical trauma, disease, biochemical and hormonal imbalances, and such physiological stimuli as physical and emotional stress.

The determination of the genetic risk in any given situation thus requires two steps. The first step is to make a precise diagnosis of the nature of the epilepsy in question. The second is to estimate the statistical probability of the occurrence of seizures in the individual at risk based upon data derived from populations of individuals with similar background—the so-called empiric risk figures.

The most clear-cut situations are those involving a single gene disorder. In the majority of such conditions, the existence of the underlying disease is evident because of the underlying biochemical defect, physical characteristics, or mental retardation. The genetic risk involves not only the risk of epilepsy but that of the related disabilities, and follows the appropriate Mendelian laws. Over a hundred clear-cut hereditary disorders which may cause epileptic seizures have been defined (see Table 20). They fall into the general categories of metabolic disorders and neurologic disorders.

General Metabolic Disorders

General metabolic disorders that may cause epilepsy include:

1. Disorders of amino acid metabolism (e.g. PKU)
2. Carbohydrate storage disorders
3. Disorders of lipid metabolism
4. Mucopolysaccharidosis
5. Disorders of vitamin metabolism (B6)

Neurologic Disorders

A number of inherited disorders of the nervous system may occasionally produce epilepsy (for example, Huntington's disease). In the inherited myoclonias (Unverricht and Lundborg), epilepsy is a common feature, although progressive dementia is a severe concomitant.

Most of the single gene diseases are rare, and together they probably account for less than 2 percent of all cases of epilepsy. However, there are two less rare dominant-inherited neurological disorders that deserve special note.

Tuberous sclerosis affects from 7,000–20,000 persons in the United States. It is inherited as a dominant trait. However, it may express itself in limited ways. In addition, it has a relatively high mutation rate; that is, there are many cases of tuberous sclerosis in which the disease appears in the offspring and neither parent is affected. The spontaneous mutation rate is from 1/60,000 to 1/120,000 per individual per generation. Tuberous sclerosis is an important cause of infantile spasms and myoclonic astatic epilepsy in infancy and childhood. It may be recognized in infancy by characteristic cutaneous areas of depigmentation. In older ages, it may be recognized by the presence of multiple small firm cutaneous nodules, especially on the "butterfly" area of the cheeks.

Neurofibromatosis is a similar inherited disorder often overlooked as an underlying condition in individuals with epilepsy. It also may often be recognized by the presence of neurocutaneous manifestations in subjects as well as in apparently unaffected relatives. It occurs in 1/2,500 to 1/3,300 births.[34]

Table 20

Genetic Syndromes Associated with Seizures

As listed in McKusick (1975). An asterisk preceding an entry indicates that the particular mode of inheritance is considered quite certain.

Autosomal Dominant Phenotypes (N = 28)

*	10940	Basal cell nevus syndrome (multiple basal cell nevi, odontogenic kerato-cysts and skeletal anomalies)
*	11710	Centralopathic epilepsy
*	12120	Convulsions, benign familial neonatal
	12125	Convulsive disorder and mental retardation
*	12300	Craniometaphyseal dysplasia
*	13110	Endocrine adenomatosis, multiple
	13210	Epilepsy, photogenic
	13220	Epilepsy, primary reading
	13210	Epilepsy, reading
*	13540	Fibromatosis, gingival, with hypertrichosis
*	13630	Flynn-Aird syndrome
	14130	Hemifacial atrophy, progressive (Parry-Romberg syndrome)
*	14310	Huntington's chorea
	14480	Hyperstosis frontalis interna (Morgagni-Stewart-Morel syndrome)
*	14940	Kok disease
*	15960	Myoclonic epilepsy, Hartung type
	15970	Myoclonus and ataxia
	15980	Myoclonus, cerebellar ataxia and deafness
*	15990	Myoclonus, hereditary essential
*	16220	Neurofibromatosis
*	16235	Neuronal ceroid-lipofuscinosis, dominant or Parry type
	16395	Noonan syndrome
	17250	Photomyoclonus, diabetes mellitus, deafness, nephropathy, and cerebral dysfunction
*	17600	Porphyria, acute intermittent
*	17620	Porphyria, variegata
	18530	Sturge-Weber syndrome
	18720	Telangiectases of brain
*	19110	Tuberous (or tuberose) sclerosis
	23100	Gaucher disease type III (juvenile and adult, cerebral)
*	23325	Goldberg Syndrome
*	23420	Hallervorden and Spatz, syndrome of
	23440	"Happy Puppet" syndrome
	23500	Hemihypertrophy
*	23620	Homocystinuria
*	23690	Hydroxlysinuria
	23740	Hyper-beta-alaninemia
*	23830	Hyperglycinemia, isolated
*	23870	Hyperlysinemia

* 23930 Hyperphosphatasia with mental retardation
* 23951 Hyperprolinemia, Type II
* 24030 Hypoadrenocorticism, with hypoparathyroidism and superficial moniliasis
   24130 Hypomagnesemia, primary
* 24520 Krabbe disease (globoid cell sclerosis)
* 24540 Lactic acidosis, familial infantile
* 24680 Lipidosis, juvenile dystonic
* 24710 Lipoid proteinosis of Urbach and Wiethe (lipotroteinosis; hyalinosis cutis et mucosae)
* 24720 Lissencephaly syndrome
* 24965 Mercaptolactate-cysteine disulfiduria
   25010 Metachromatic leukodystrophy, late infantile (metachromatic leukoencephalopathy; metachromatic form of diffuse cerebral sclerosis; sulfatide lipidosis)
* 25090 Methionine malabsorption syndrome
   25240 Mucolipidosis I (lipomucopolysaccharidosis)
* 25250 Mucolipidosis II (I-cell disease)
* 25480 Myoclonic epilepsy of Unverricht and Lundberg
* 25660 Neuoroaxonal dystrophy, infantile (Seitelberger)
* 25673 Neuronal ceroid-lipofuscinosis, infantile Finnish type
* 25720 Niemann-Pick disease (sphingomyelin lipidosis)
* 26160 Phenylketonuria
   26440 Pseudohypoparathyroidism, Type II
* 26610 Pyridoxine dependency with seizures
   27000 Sidbury syndrome
* 27060 Spastic diplegia, infantile type
   27255 Tachycardia, hypertension, microphthalmos, hyperglycinuria
* 27289 Tay-Sachs disease: GM2-gangliosidosis, Type I
   27890 Xylosidase deficiency

Autosomal Recessive Phenotypes (N = 66)

   20360 Alopecia-epilepsy-oligophrenia syndrome of Moynahan (Familial congenital alopecia, epilepsy, mental retardation and unusual EEG)
* 20370 Alpers' diffuse degeneration of cerebral gray matter (poliodystrophia cerebri progressiva) with hepatic cirrhosis
* 20420 Amaurotic family idiocy, juvenile type (Batten disease in England, Vogt-Spielmeyer disease on the continent)
* 20430 Amaurotic idiocy, adult type (Kuf disease)
* 20440 Amaurotic idiocy, congenital form
* 20460 Amaurotic idiocy, late infantile, with multilamellar cytosomes
* 20657 Angiomatosis, diffuse cortico-meningeal, of Divry and VanBogaert
* 20780 Argininemia
* 20790 Argininosuccinicaciduria
   20870 Ataxia with myoclonus epilepsy and presenile dementia
* 21220 Carnosinemia
   21340 Cerebello-parenchymal disorder V (Spinodentate atrophy: Dyssynergia cerebellaris myoclonica of Hunt)

	21360	Cerebral calcification, non-arteriosclerotic
	21380	Cerebral gigantism (Sotos syndrome)
*	21570	Citrullinuria (citrullinemia)
	21720	Convulsive disorder, familial, with prenatal or early onset
	21790	Cornelia de Lange syndrome
*	21800	Corpus callosum, agenesis of
*	21830	Craniodiaphyseal dysplasia
*	21890	Crome syndrome
*	21950	Cystathioninuria
	22030	Deaf-mutism and familial myoclonus epilepsy
*	22050	Deaf-mutism and onychodystrophy
*	22180	Dermo-chondro-corneal dystrophy of Francois
	22440	Dysostosis, enchondral, of Nierhoff-Huber type
	22680	Epilepsy, photogenic, with spastic diplegia and mental retardation
*	22905	Folic acid, transport defect involving
*	22950	Fructose and galactose intolerance
*	22960	Fructose intolerance, hereditary (fructosemia)
*	23040	Galactosemia

X-linked Phenotypes (N = 10)

	30190	Borjeson syndrome (mental deficiency, epilepsy, endocrine disorders)
	30410	Corpus callosum, partial agenesis of
*	30760	Hypomagnesemic tetany
*	30800	Hypoxanthine guanine phosphoribosyl transferase deficiency (Lesch-Nyhan syndrome)
*	30940	Menkes syndrome (kinky hair disease)
*	30950	Mental deficiency (Martin-Bell, or Renpenning type)
	30965	Methylmandelicaciduria
*	31140	Paine syndrome (microcephaly with spastic diplegia)
	31145	Pallister W syndrome
*	31160	Pelizaeus-Merzbacher disease

Magnitude of Genetic Risk

In the majority of persons with epilepsy no clear-cut inherited disease can be demonstrated, and counseling must rely upon empiric risk figures for the actual subgroup of the individual patient. The following data are presented to indicate the order of magnitude of the genetic risks involved in various situations.

What Are the Chances that an Affected Parent Will Have a Child Subject to Epilepsy? For unexplained reasons, taking epilepsy as a whole, the likelihood that an affected mother will have an affected child is greater than that an affected father will. In fact, in the series shown in Table 21 the risk for epileptic fathers was little greater than that within the general population.

Data are not available for specific types of epilepsy according to which

Table 21

Epilepsy in Offspring of Epileptic Parents

Reference	Control	Affected Parent Mother	Father
Annegers et al., 1976	0.6	2.8%	0
Tsuboi and Endo, 1977		2.9%	1.7%

Table 22

Frequency of Epilepsy in Offspring of
Epileptic Parents According to Seizure Type

Author	Type of Seizure or Epilepsy	% of Offspring with Seizures
Alstrom, 1950	Combined	2.7*
Harvald, 1958	Combined	1.7
Thom & Walker, 1922	Combined	7.7
Stein, 1933	Combined	2.2
Tsuboi & Endo, 1977	Combined	9.1
Tsuboi & Endo, 1977	Tonic-clonic	9.2
Tsuboi & Christian, 1973	Impulsive petit mal	13.6
Anderman, 1972	Focal-surgical cases	3.6
Tsuboi & Endo, 1977	Complex partial	8.9
Tsuboi & Endo, 1977	Focal	5.9
Alstrom, 1950	Seizures of known etiology	1.6*
Alstrom, 1950	Seizures of unknown etiology	3.1

*Excludes offspring having single seizure only.

parent is affected (Table 22). Combining both parents, there is a 6 percent risk for the children of parents with idiopathic (primary generalized) epilepsy, compared to a 1.6 percent risk for "symptomatic" epilepsy. The latter figure probably differs little from that of the general population. It should be noted that in these estimates, the "control" figure is *not* the 1 percent figure of the general prevalence of epilepsy, but is a cumulative figure for the occurrence of epilepsy at any stage of the subject's lifetime. This figure is 1 percent by age 20, 1.7 percent by age 40, and 3.3 percent by age 80.[35]

Given that One Child Has Epilepsy, What Is the Risk for Subsequent

Children? Theoretically, the risk for subsequent children should be approximately the same as the risk of an affected child when one parent is affected. Some data are available for various types of epilepsy (Table 23). However, these data are contaminated because in some instances febrile seizures are included as "epilepsy." Since 3-5 percent of children experience at least one febrile seizure, their inclusion will greatly inflate the risk figure. In other instances, siblings, parents, and grandparents are lumped, and it is not possible to separate out the siblings. Finally, many studies fail to provide data on a control population and thus provide no indication of the comparative risk for the person with epilepsy unless one uses the general figure cited above.

Table 23

Frequency of Epilepsy in Siblings of Persons
with Epilepsy by Seizure Type

Author	Type Seizure or Epilepsy	% of Siblings with Seizures
Alstrom, 1950	Combined	1.5
Harvald, 1954	Combined	3.4
Kimball, 1954	Combined	9.5
Metrakos & Metrakos, 1960	Combined	9.6
Ounstead, 1952	Combined	4.1
Van den Berg, 1974	Combined	6.6
Metrakos & Metrakos, 1961	With centrencephalic EEG	13.5
Matthes, 1969	Pyknolepsy	3.7
Doose et al., 1973	Absence with spike-wave EEG	7.0
Degen, 1972	Infantile spasm	4.5
Doose, 1970	Myoclonic astatic	12.6
Matthes, 1969	Myoclonic astatic	3.1
Vogel, 1969	Myoclonic akinetic	12.6
Tsuboi & Christian, 1973	Impulsive petit mal	5.4
Anderman, 1972	Focal-surgical cases	1.3
Gerkin et al., 1977	Partial with focal spike EEG	1.9
Muller et al., 1973	Focal	3.5
Jensen, 1975	Complex partial (temporal lobe)	2.9
Lindsay, 1971	Complex partial	15.0
Lindsay, 1971	Complex partial with previous status	30.0
Lindsay, 1971	Complex partial with known injury	1.9
Alstrom, 1950	Unknown etiology	1.6
Alstrom, 1950	Known etiology	1.3

In general, the risk of epilepsy in the sibling of a child with primary generalized epilepsy, whether tonic-clonic, absence, or myoclonic, was between 3-7 percent. For those with infantile spasms or myoclonic astatic (secondary generalized) epilepsy, the figure is 5-10 percent.

For the partial epilepsies the figure is lower, running 1.3–3.5 percent and thus barely exceeding the control level.

The above figures indicate that in those families within which only a single member is affected with epilepsy, even in instances of primary generalized epilepsy, the risk for siblings, while two to three times that of the general population, is still under 10 percent, while for the symptomatic (partial) epilepsies it barely exceeds that of the general population.

However, it has been possible to define certain high-risk situations in which a combination of factors is operative or where several family members are affected. The variables which have been studied are (1) type of epilepsy—primary generalized is associated with increased risk; (2) presence of photoconvulsive EEG—which increases risk; (3) number of affected relatives; and (4) myoclonic seizures. The highest risks are as follows: (1) one child and both parents affected—risk for sibling 33.3 percent; (2) child with photoconvulsive epilepsy—risk for sibling 30.8 percent; (3) child with single seizure and one parent affected—risk for sibling 6.8-13.5 percent.[36]

The multifactorial nature of epileptic inheritance is most strikingly demonstrated in studies comparing monozygotic and dizygotic twins (Table 24). For primary generalized epilepsies, these studies show 80-100 percent concordance for monozygotic twins, compared to 4-5 percent for dizygotics. Other studies,[37] especially those relying on the study of EEG findings in relatives of persons with epilepsy, indicate that an inheritable epileptic predisposition is more widespread than is the overt seizure (see Table 12).

Table 24

Concordance for Epilepsy in Twins

Author	Type Epilepsy	% Affected by Type Twin	
		Monozygotic	Dizygotic
Gedda & Tatarelli, 1971	Idiopathic	97	15
Braconi, 1962	Idiopathic	91	50
	Symptomatic	62	14
Conrad, 1935	Idiopathic	86	4
	Acquired	13	0
Lennox, 1947	Etiology unknown	83	6
	Etiology known	16	0

Conclusion

In general, epilepsy carries a small but significant genetic risk for the child of a woman with epilepsy or the sibling of an epileptic child. This risk is greatest in the primary generalized epilepsies, and especially those with myoclonic and photosensitive features. Where several members of the family are affected, the risk is significantly increased. Genetic counseling requires a thorough evaluation of the subject and family and cannot be undertaken lightly.

REFERENCES

1. Gastaut, H.: Dictionary of Epilepsy. World Health Organization, Geneva, 1973.
2. Engel, J., Jr., Wolfson, L. and Brown, L.: Anatomical correlates of electrical and behavioral events related to amygdaloid kindling. *Ann. Neurol.*, 3:538-544, 1978.
3. Vosu, H. and Wise, R. A.: Cholinergic seizure kindling in the rat. comparison of caudate, amygdala and hippocampus. *Behav. Biol.* 13:491-495, 1975.
4. Willmore, L. J., Sypert, G. W., Munsen, J. B. and Hurd, R. W.: Chronic focal epileptogenic discharges inducted by injection of iron into rat and cat cortex. *Science*, 200:1501-1502, 1978.
5. Noebels, J. L. and Sidman, R. L.: Inherited epilepsy: Spke-wave and focal motor seizures in the mutant mouse tottering. *Science*, 204:1334-1336, 1979.
6. Daly, D. D.: Ictal manifestations of complex partial seizures. In: J. K. Penry and D. D. Daly (ed.), *Advances in Neurology*, Vol. II, Complex Partial Seizures and Their Treatment, N.Y.: Raven Press, 1975, p. 57-83.
7. Jeavons, P. M.: Nosological problems of myoclonic epilepsies of childhood and adolescence. *Dev. Med. Child Neurol.*, 19:3-8, 1977.
8. Beaussart, M. and Faou, R.: Evolution of epilepsy with rolandic paroxysmal foci: A study of 324 cases. *Epilepsia*, 19:337-342, 1978.
9. Seki, T., Kawahara, Y., and Hirose, M.: The long term prognosis of infantile spasms. The present condition of cases of infantile spasms followed in school age. *Folia Psychiat. Neurol. Jap.*, 30:279-306, 1976.
10. Aicardi, J.: Course and prognosis of certain childhood epilepsies with predominantly myoclonic seizures. Proceedings, 10th International Epilepsy Symposium, Vancouver, Sept. 10, 1978.
11. Annegers, J. F., Hauser, W. A., Elveback, L. R., and Kurland, L. T.: The risk of epilepsy following febrile convulsions. *Neurology*, 29:297-303, 1979.
12. Seki et al., op. cit.
13. Woodbury, L.: Incidence and prevalence of seizure disorders including the epilepsies in the U.S.A. In: The Commission for the Control of Epilepsy and Its Consequences, DHEW (NIH) Pub. #78-279, Vo. IV, p. 24-106, 1978.
14. Metrakos, K. and Metrakos, J. D.: Genetics of convulsive disorders. II. Genetics and EEG studies in centrencephalic epilepsy. *Neurology*, 11:474-483, 1961.
15. Metrakos, J. D.: Genetics of Epilepsy. In: P. J. Vinkin and G. W. Bruyn (ed.), *Handbook of Clinical Neurology*. Elsevier, N.Y. Vol. 15, 1974, p. 429-439. J. D. Metrakos, K. Metrakos. Genetic Studies in Clinical Epilepsy. In: H. H. Jasper, A. A. Ward, Jr., A. Pope (ed.), *Basic Mechanisms of the Epilepsies*. Boston: Little, Brown, 1969.
16. Hauser, A.: EEG Findings in a Defined Population of Persons with Epilepsy. Rochester, Minn. 1979. Unpublished data.
17. Gastaut, H. and Gastaut, J. L.: Computerized transverse axial tomography in epilepsy. *Epilepsia*, 17:325-336, 1976.

18. Commission for the control of epilepsy and its consequences. *The CAT Scan*, Vol. II, part 2, p. 323-329, 1978.
19. Hauser, W. A., Schwanebeck, E. M., Churn, M. M., and Anderson, V. E.: Seizure recurrence following 'Single Seizures.' *Neurology* 29:578, 1979.
20. Blom, S., Heijbel, J., and Bergfors, P. G.: Incidence of epilepsy in children: A follow-up study 3 years after the first seizure. *Epilepsia*, 19:343-350, 1978.
21. Wada, J., Sato, M., Wok, A., Green, V. P., and Troupin, A. S.: Prophylactic effects of phenytoin, phenobarbital and carbamazepine examined in kindling cat preparation. *Arch. Neurol.* 33:426-434, 1976.
22. Leahy, W. R. and Freeman, J. M.: Status epilepticus. In: Commission for the Control of Epilepsy and Its Consequences, DHEW (NIH) 78-311, Vol. II, Part 1, p. 163-174, 1978.
23. Green L. W. and Roter, D.: The literature on patient compliance and implications for cost-effective patient education programs in epilepsy. Commission for the Control of Epilepsy and Its Consequences, Vol. II, Part I, p. 391-417, 1978.
24. Iivanianen, M., Viukari, M. and Helle, E. P.: Cerebellar atrophy in phenytoin-treated mentally retarded epileptics. *Epilepsia*, 18:375-385, 1977.
25. Falconer, M. and Davidson, S.: Coarse features in epilepsy as a consequence of anticonvulsant therapy. *Lancet*, 2:1112-1114, 1973.
26. Li, F. P., Willar, D. C., Goodman, R., and Vorster, G.: Malignant lymphoma after F.P.H. treatment. *Cancer*, 36:1359-1362, 1975. Sorrell, T. C. and Forbes, I. J.: Phenytoin sensitivity in a case of phenytoin associated Hodgkin's disease. *Australian, N.Z. Jour. Med.*, 5:144-147, 1975.
27. Suchy, F. J., Balisteri, W. F., Buchino, J. J., Sondheimer, J. M., Bates, S. R., Kearns, G. L., Stull, J. D., and Bove, K. E.: Acute hepatic failure associated with use of sodium valproate. *New England J. Med.*, 300:962-966, 1979.
28. Rasmussen, T.: Cortical resection in the treatment of focal epilepsy. In: D. P. Purpura, J. K. Penry, R. D. Walter (ed.), *Advances in Neurology*, Vol. 8, Neurosurgical Management of the Epilepsies. N.Y.: Raven Press, 1975, p. 139-154; Rayport, M.: Role of Neurosurgery in the management of medication-refractory epilepsy. In: Commission for the Control of Epilepsy and Its Consequences, DHEW (NIH) 78-311, Vol. II, Part I, 1978 pp. 314-343.
29. Jensen, I.: Temporal lobe epilepsy: On whom to operate and when. In: J. K. Penry (ed.), *Epilepsy. The Eighth International Symposium*. New York: Raven, 1977, pp. 325-331.
30. Nelson, K. B. and Ellenberg, J. H.: Prognosis in children with febrile convulsions. *Pediatrics*, 61:720-727, 1978. Annegers, J. F., Hauser, W. A., and Elveback, L. R.: Remission and relapse of seizures in patients with epilepsy. *Epilepsia*, 1979 20:729-737.
31. Wolf, S. M., Carr, A., Davis, D. C., Davidson, S., Dale, E. P., Forsythe, A., Goldenberg, E. D., Hanson, R., Lulejian, G. A., Nelson, M. A., Treitman, P., and Weinstein, A.: The value of phenobarbital in the child who has had a single febrile seizure: A controlled prospective study. *Pediatrics*, 59:378-385, 1977.
32. Thorn, I.: Prophylactic treatment of febrile convulsions with continuous phenobarbital contra intermittant diazepam. *Dev. Med. Child Neurol.*, 22:267-268, 1980. Knudsen, F. U. and Vestermark, S. Prophylactic diazepam or phenobarbitone in febrile convulsions: A prospective controlled study. *Arch. Dis. Child.* 53:660-663, 1978.
33. Metrakos, J. D.: Genetic counseling. In: Report of the commission for the control of epilepsy and its consequences, DHEW (NIH) 78-311, Vol. II, Part I, 1978, p. 175-215; Anderson, V. E.: Genetic counseling for epilepsy. In: Report of the Commission for the Control of Epilepsy and Its Consequences, DHEW (NIH) 78-311, Vol. II, Part 1, 1978, p. 141-162.
34. Crowe, F. W., Schull, W. J., and Neil, J. W.: A clinical pathological and genetic study of multiple neurofibromatosis. Springfield, IL: Charles Thomas, 1956.
35. Anderson, V. E., op. cit.; Woodbury, L., op. cit.
36. Hauser, W. A., Chern, M. M., Anderson, V. E., and Mayersdorf, A.: Seizure history in families—Factors affecting sibling risk for seizures. Proceedings from Ep. Int'l Symposium, Vancouver, Sept. 10-14, 1978.

37. Metrakos, J. D. and Metrakos, K.: Genetic studies in clinical epilepsy. In: H. H. Jasper, A. A. Ward, J. & A. Pope (eds.), *Basic Mechanisms of the Epilepsies*. Boston: Little, Brown, 1969, pp. 700-708.

TABLE REFERENCES

Table 1. Abstracted from: Merlis, J. K. Proposal for an International Classification of the Epilepsies. Epilepsia 11:114-119, 1970.

Table 2. Eva D. Anderman, 1972. Focal Epilepsy and Related Disorders. Thesis. McGill Univ.

Table 3. Abstracted from: Gastaut, H. Clinical and electroencephalographical classification of epileptic seizures. Epilepsia 11:102-113, 1970.

Figure 1. Results of Electrical Stimulation of the Cerebral Cortex After Foerster from Bailey, P. Intracranial Tumors, Thomas, 1933.

Table 4. Unpublished Data. R. L. Masland and W. S. Lockhart, Jr.

Table 5. Ibid.

Table 6. Commission for the Control of Epilepsy and Its Consequences, Vol. 1, p. 25 (Woodbury, 1978); Vol. IV, p. 107-114 (Woodbury, 1978).

Table 7. Commission for the Control of Epilepsy and Its Consequences, Woodbury, 1978 (Vol. IV, p. 100).

Table 8. M. Rutter, P. Graham & W. Yule, 1970. A Neuropsychiatric Study in Childhood. In: *Clinics of Developmental Medicine* #35/36 Lippincott; P. D. Denneril, E. A. Rodin, S. Gonzalez, 1966. Neurological and Psychological Factors Related to Employability of Persons with Epilepsy. Epilepsia 7:318-29.

Table 9. H. L. Shapiro and E. A. Rodin, 1978. Seizure Frequency of Persons with Major and Minor Seizures, in Report of the Commission for the Control of Epilepsy and Its Consequences, Vol. I, p. 22.

Table 10. E. A. Rodin, H. L. Shapiro, and K. Lennox, 1976. *Epilepsy and Life Performance*. Lafayette Clinic, Detroit.

Table 11. Commission for the Control of Epilepsy and its Consequences, 1978.

Table 12. Metrakos and Metrakos, 1961.

Table 13. Gastaut and Gastaut, 1976.

Table 14. Blom et al., 1978.

Table 15. E. van der Kleijn, T. Vree, P. Gallen, F. Shobten, H. Westenberg, Kinetics of Drug Interaction. In: The Treatment of Epilepsy, International Journal Clin. Pharmacol. 16:467-473.

Table 16. H. Kutt, Diphenylhydantoin. Interactions with other drugs in man, in Woodbury, D. M., Penry, J. K., and Schmidt, R. P. Eds. Antiepileptic Drugs. P. 169-180. Raven Press N.Y. 1972.

Table 17. Tri-state Epilepsy Association, Inc. Evansville, Indiana 47711

Table 18. J. W. Hansen & N. C. Myrianthopoulos, 1976. Risks to the Offspring of Women Treated With Hydantoin Anticonvulsants, With Emphasis on the Fetal Hydantoin Syndrome. J. Ped. 89:662-668; G. H. Visser, H. J. Huisjes, and J. Elshone, 1976. Anticonvulsants and Fetal Malformation. Lancet, 1976, 1:970.

L. Dansky, E. Andermann, P. M. Loughman & J. E. Gibbons 1977. Congenital malformations in Offspring of Epileptic women: A Clinical Investigation of teratogenic effects of Anticonvulsant Medication. Epilepsia 18:284.

Y. Biale, H. Lewenthal, & N. B. Aderet 1975. Congenital Malformation due to Anticonvulsant Drugs. O. Gyn 45:439-442.

J. G. Koppe, W. Bosman, V. M. Oppers, F. Spaans, & G. J. Kloosterman 1973. Epilepsy and Congenital Malformation. Nederlands Tijdschrift Voor Geneeskunde 117:220-224.

Table 20. Based in part on a list prepared by Roswell Eldridge, M.D. (IR, NINCDS, NIH). V. McKusick 1975. Mendelian Inheritance in Man. Johns Hopkins University Press. Baltimore.

Table 21. J. F. Annegers, W. A. Hauser, L. R. Elveback, V. E. Anderson, & L. T. Kurland, 1976. Seizure Disorders in Offspring of Parents with a History of Seizures—A Maternal-Paternal Difference? Epilepsia 17:1-9.

T. Tsuboi & S. Endo, 1977. Incidence of Seizures and EEG Abnormalities Among Offspring of Epileptic Patients. Hum. Genetik 36:173-189.

Table 22. C. H. Alstrom, 1950. A Study of Epilepsy in its Clinical, Social and Genetic Aspects. Arta Psychiat. Copenhagen 63:1-284.

B. Harvald, 1958. Hereditary Factors in Epilepsy. Med. Clin. North Am. 58:345-348.

D. A. Thom & G. S. Walker, 1922. Epilepsy in the Offspring of Epileptics. Am. J. Psychiatr. 1:613-627.

C. Stein, 1933. Hereditary Factors in Epilepsy. A Comparative Study of 1000 Institutionalized Epileptics and 1115 Non-epileptic Controls. Am. J. Psychiat. 12:989-1037.

Tsuboi, Endo, 1977. (Referenced with Table 21)

T. Tsuboi & W. Christian, 1973. On the Genetics of the Primary Generalized Epilepsy with Sporadic Myoclonias of Impulsive Petit Mal Type. Humangenetic 19:155-182.

E. D. Anderman, 1972. Focal Epilepsy and Related Disorders. Thesis, McGill Univ.

Table 23. Alstrom '50 (Table 22); Harvald '58 (Table 22); Kimball, O. P. On the inheritance of epilepsy. Wisc. Med. J., 1954 53:271-276; Metrakos, K. & Metrakos J. D., 1960. Genetics of Convulsive Disorders. I. Introduction, Problems, Methods, and Base Lines. Neurology 10:228-240.

C. Ounstead, 1952. The Factor of Inheritance in Convulsive Disorders in Childhood. Proc. Roy. Soc. Med. 45:37-40.

B. J. van den Berg, 1974. Studies on Convulsive Disorders in Young Children. IV Incidence of Convulsions among Siblings. Dev. Med. Child Neurol. 16:457-464.

Metrakos & Metrakos, 1961 (Ref. 14).

A. Matthes, 1969. Genetic Studies in Epilepsy. In H. Gastaut, H. Jasper, J. Bancaud and A. Wattregny, Eds. The Physiopathogenesis of the Epilepsies. CC Thomas, Springfield.

H. Doose, H. Gerkin, T. Horstmann & E. Volzke 1973. Genetic Factors in Spike-Wave Absences. Epilepsia 14:57-75.

R. Degen, 1972. Probleme der Atiologie und EKG der kindlichen Epilepsie. Dtsch. Ges. Wesen. 27:71-76.

H. Doose, H. Gerkin, R. Lemhardt, E. Volzke and C. Volz, 1970. Centrencephalic Myoclonic-Astatis Petit Mal Clinical and Genetic Investigations. Neuropediatrie 2:59-78.

F. Vogel, 1969. The EEG of Genetically Different Types of Inherited Myoclonic Epilepsy. EEG Clin Neurophysiol. 26:444.

Tsuboi, Christian (Table 22).

Anderman, 1972 (Table 22).

H. Gerkin, R. Kiefer, H. Doose and E. Volzke, 1977. Genetic Factors in Childhood Epilepsy with Focal Sharp Waves. Neuropaediatrie 8:3-9.

K. Muller, H. Arnold, B. Bruhn, 1973. Familial Predisposition in Focal Epilepsy. Schw. Arch-Neurol. Neuropsychiat. 113:45-55.

I. Jensen, 1975. Genetic Factors in Temporal Lobe Epilepsy. Acta Neurol. Scand. 52:281-394.

J. M. M. Lindsay, 1971. Genetics and Epilepsy: a Model from Critical Path Analysis. Epilepsia 12:47-54.

Table 24. L. Gedda and R. Tatarelli, 1971. Essential Isochronic Epilepsy in Monozygotic Twin Pairs. Acta Genet. Med. 20:380-383.

L. Braconi, 1962. Twin Research in Epilepsy. Acta Genet. 11:138-157.

W. Conrad, 1935. Erbanlage und Epilepsie. Untersuchungen an einer Serie von 253 Zwillingspaaren. Z. Neurol. Psychiat. 153:271-326.

W. G. Lennox, 1947. Sixty-Six Twin Pairs Affected by Seizures. Assoc. Res. Ner. & Ment. Dis. Proc. 26:11-34.

2

THE TREATMENT OF SEIZURES: SPECIAL PSYCHOTHERAPEUTIC AND PSYCHOBIOLOGICAL TECHNIQUES

DANIEL T. WILLIAMS, M.D.

The clinical literature on epilepsy contains many references to the role of environmental stress and emotional experiences as precipitants of seizures.[1] Several workers have reported emotional activation of the electroencephalogram in patients with convulsive disorders, particularly those with psychomotor and sensory epilepsy.[2] Allen reported that 42 of 182 cases (23.1 percent) of patients with neurologically diagnosed seizure disorders were found to have emotional factors related to the occurrence of seizures.[3] Mignone et al. note that 53 percent of their 151 patients who had unequivocally positive EEGs reported precipitation of seizures by stress.[4] Furthermore, the direct emotional activation of seizures has been documented with pentylenetetrazol treated mice,[5] in genetically susceptible dogs,[6] and in alumina cream epileptic rhesus monkeys,[7] when these animals were exposed to various forms of environmental stress.

It therefore seems reasonable to posit that psychotherapy and related techniques that enable the patient and his or her family to deal more effectively with the emotional trauma of uncontrolled seizures, as well as with other environmental and intrapsychic stresses, could be helpful adjunctive aids in psychological and hence neurophysiological stabilization. In this way, psychotherapeutic and related psychobiological techniques can sometimes contribute to breaking the cycle of repetitive, seizure-inducing psychophysiological activation that appears to occur in some patients whose seizures are not controlled by medication alone.[8]

The author gratefully acknowledges the assistance of Dr. David Mostofsky in the preparation of this chapter.

Differential Diagnosis for
Psychotherapeutic/Psychobiological Intervention

The clinical importance of determining the specific type of seizure disorder has been noted in Chapter 1. Differential diagnosis is also important in determining the possible merits of psychotherapeutic intervention with seizure patients. The most crucial distinction to make in this regard is between primary neurogenic seizures and those which are exclusively or primarily of psychological origin, although it should be noted that there are important subdivisions of and possible areas of overlap between these two major categories.

Neurogenic Seizures

The various types of neurogenic seizures have been discussed in Chapter 1. As will be seen below, especially in the case of sensory-precipitated seizures, the particular type of neurogenic seizure may be relevant in determining the particular type of psychotherapeutic/psychobiological control strategy which is appropriate.

With any type of neurogenic seizure disorder it is important in the course of history taking and clinical assessment to determine, insofar as possible, to what extent emotional factors may play a role in precipitating the seizures. Moreover, the mental health practitioner should be constantly attuned to the possible role of psychogenic precipitants of neurogenic seizures in his or her ongoing contact with the patient and the patient's family.

Psychogenic Seizures

With the advent of the third edition of the Diagnostic and Statistical Manual of Mental Disorders (DSM-III), recently published by the American Psychiatric Association,[9] seizures or seizure-like phenomena of primarily psychological origin are now most usefully subdivided into the following categories:

1. *Factitious Seizures.* Factitious disorders are characterized by physical or psychological symptoms that are produced by the patient and are under the patient's voluntary control. The judgment that a particular piece of behavior is under voluntary control is made by exclusion after all involuntary mechanisms for the behavior have been considered.
   a. *Purposeful Medication Noncompliance.* A patient whose seizures have previously been controlled with anticonvulsant medication in the therapeutic range may be found at the time of uncontrolled seizures to

have a markedly subtherapeutic or absent serum anticonvulsant level. Missing a single dose or two of medication might be accidental rather than intentional. A marked fall in serum anticonvulsant level, however, in the face of the patient's report of taking the medication as prescribed, would justify an inference of voluntary production of illness.[10] (A variation on this theme would be a patient who becomes "toxic" by purposely ingesting excessive amounts of anticonvulsant medication.)

   b. *Feigned Seizures With No Apparent Goal.* A person who purposely feigned having a seizure with no apparent goal other than to assume the role of a patient would also be considered as having a factitious seizure disorder. This would be true whether or not there existed a concomitant bona fide neurogenic seizure disorder. The presence of such a factitious disorder is usually symptomatic of a severe underlying personality disturbance.

2. *Somatoform Disorders.* This term denotes a group of disorders that suggest organic illness for which there are no organic findings to explain the symptoms and for which there is positive evidence that the symptoms are linked to psychological factors. As with factitious illness and malingering, a somatoform disorder may coexist with a true neurogenic seizure disorder. Unlike factitious illness or malingering, the symptom production in somatoform disorders is not under voluntary control. That is, the patient does not have conscious awareness of controlling production or withdrawal of the symptoms.

   a. *Somatization Disorder (Briquet's Syndrome).* This is a chronic but fluctuating disorder which begins early in life and is characterized by recurrent and multiple somatic complaints for which medical attention is sought but which are not apparently due to any physical illness. Anxiety and depressive features are common. In addition, abuse of alcohol and other drugs and diverse forms of antisocial behavior are frequently encountered. This syndrome is more common in women. It may include the presence of conversion seizures and is often associated with a histrionic personality disorder.

   b. *Conversion (Hysterical) Seizures.* These symptoms have traditionally been explained as serving the purpose of reducing conflict-generated anxiety by keeping the conflict out of awareness while at the same time permitting it to be expressed symbolically. Conversion seizures usually develop in a setting of severe psychological stress. Yet the patient may display "la belle indifférence," reflecting a relative lack of concern in view of the seriousness of the symptom. This feature of apparent calmness may be of dubious diagnostic value, however, since it is not always present with conversion seizures, and it may be present in patients with neurogenic seizures who are stoical about their situation.

3. *Malingering.* Here, seizures are consciously and voluntarily feigned. Moreover, this is done in pursuit of a goal which, when known, is obviously recognizable with an understanding of the individual's circumstances. Examples of this type of goal would include avoiding work or military service, obtaining financial compensation, evading criminal prosecution, and obtaining drugs.

Characteristics of Psychogenic Seizures

The following characteristics may be delineated as favoring a diagnosis of "seizure-like phenomena" under the various categories outlined above, as distinct from true neurogenic seizures:[11]

1. The seizures emerge under stressful circumstances with an apparent primary gain of anxiety alleviation.
2. There are secondary gains, such as getting attention, being excused from work, collecting financial compensation, or escaping from an intolerable social situation.
3. There are other conversion symptoms and/or histrionic personality features.
4. The patient is hypnotizable and can recall the details of the seizure under hypnosis.[12]
5. The seizures fail to conform to a physiologic pattern.
6. There is generally no incontinence during the attack, and after the attack, one observes none of the drowsiness or depression of either stretch reflexes or oculovestibular (caloric) response that characterizes most epilepsy.
7. The tongue is rarely bitten, and the patient does not generally injure him or herself.
8. Corneal reflexes are present and plantar reflexes are flexor.
9. The EEG during the seizure is normal and shows no post-ictal slowing.

The more of the above criteria which are met, the greater the likelihood that a "seizure-like phenomenon" rather than a true neurogenic seizure occurred. Further, it should be noted that some of these criteria are more discriminating than others, with EEG monitoring during the seizure being most specific, if it can be obtained.[13]

Diagnostic Difficulties

It should be noted that even the experienced psychotherapist may encounter difficulty in ascertaining the level of the patient's awareness of relevant psychodynamic issues leading to a "seizure-like episode."[14]

Additionally, it may be impossible for the clinician, even when observing a given seizure, to be certain about the distinction between a "seizure-like episode" and a psychogenically precipitated neurogenic seizure, unless there is the benefit of ongoing EEG monitoring. This is especially true when a psychomotor (partial complex) seizure is in question, because the presentation may be so atypical.[15]

Finally, just as any of the various subtypes of psychogenic seizures may occur in a patient with a coexisting neurogenic seizure disorder, so also different forms of psychogenic seizures may occur in the same patient over time. The above categories may therefore be most usefully thought of as part of a spectrum of possible but not necessarily mutually exclusive psychopathological determinants of seizures.

Epidemiological Considerations

Few epidemiological studies have attempted to distinguish emotionally based "seizure-like phenomena" from neurogenic seizures, probably owing to the difficulties in differential diagnosis outlined above. In a group of 469 navy personnel admitted to the hospital because of seizures, Rossen[16] found that 209, or 44 percent, were not epileptic, as judged by criteria available at that time. Other studies in the armed forces have yielded similar results.[17] Clearly there is a need for further research in this area with the more sophisticated diagnostic methods currently available, such as ongoing EEG cassette monitoring.[18]

OVERVIEW OF PSYCHOTHERAPEUTIC/ PSYCHOBIOLOGICAL TREATMENT STRATEGIES

With all the emphasis that has been placed on the importance of differential diagnosis above, one might anticipate that there would be a clear correlation between specific seizure type and specific psychotherapeutic treatment strategy to be proposed. For the most part, however, this is not so. Rather, the focus on diagnosis is geared primarily to emphasize the fact that the treatment of choice for a patient with uncontrolled seizures may not be simply an increase of dose or change of type of anticonvulsant medication. Instead, in selected instances, it may be to address the sources of environmental or intrapsychic stress which are the crux of the problem. Unfortunately, such issues are often addressed only after multiple medication regimens have been tried and have failed. The mental health professional is then called in as the last hope in a state of crisis or desperation. While this situation may appeal to a therapist with dramatic rescue fantasies, it would clearly be better for the patient if important psychogenic features of his or her uncontrolled seizures were recognized and dealt with earlier. In those settings where there is a good liaison relationship between the neurologist and the mental health professional, the prospects for such earlier collaborative effort are improved.

A broad spectrum of techniques that are part of the general armamentarium of both dynamically and behaviorally trained practitioners have been applied to the control of seizure disorders. The studies are outlined in a format delineated by Mostofsky and Balaschak.[19] It is, however, extremely difficult, if not impossible, to examine any one psychotherapeutic procedure independent of other overlapping or concurrent therapeutic influences. In part this is because the environmental and intrapsychic triggers of seizures are often complex and multidetermined, so that treatment programs are commonly designed to attack more than a single objective. In fact, almost all studies cited below implicitly or explicitly combine more than a single category of procedure in a given therapy program.

The treatment strategies below have been grouped under the headings of Conditioning Techniques, Psychodynamic Approaches, Relaxation and Hypnosis, and Biofeedback. Reports are cited to illustrate the diversity of behavioral and psychodynamic approaches that have been reported to be successfully applied in the treatment of seizure disorders. Each of the references cited describes either one or a few cases in which the particular strategy applied led to improved seizure control as compared to pre-treatment baseline frequency. It should be noted that reports describing both neurogenic and psychogenic seizures are included. Individual reports are not always rigorous in distinguishing between neurogenic and psychogenic seizures, nor in controlling for possible effects of unreported medication changes. Further, reports involving both adults and children are mentioned.

Conditioning Techniques

Conditioning techniques include denial of reward, penalty program, relief (avoidance) punishment, overt and covert rewards, and habituation (extinction).

Denial of Reward

Attentive concern toward the patient may tend to positively reinforce seizures. Thus the reward denial paradigm requires that the occurrence of a seizure is not followed by a display of care, concern, or indeed any attention. The seizure is ignored, as one might ignore some other undesirable behavior such as a tantrum. The expectation is that continued nonrecognition of this behavior will lead to its extinction.

Gardner[20] describes the treatment of a 10-year-old girl with psychogenic seizures using this approach. After two weeks, seizures dropped from six to eight per week to zero. When the parents started paying attention to inappropriate behavior again, seizures resumed. When treatment was reinstituted, seizures stopped again. A year later, the patient was still seizure-free.

Penalty Program

In the penalty program, when the patient has a seizure he or she is asked to enter a "time-out room" or equivalent environment in which he or she does not have access to reinforcement. As contrasted to the "denial of reward" category, this approach, rather than passive ignoring of the behavior, required that the observer intervene and react to the patient. In an institutional setting, this may involve moving a patient from an open ward to a less open setting or denying the patient visits or off-ground privileges. In a home or school setting with a child, this might entail denying the child a recess period or another favorite activity. It is explained to the patient that such action is being taken so that he or she will no longer be in danger, and that he or she will be able to return to previous activities when his or her condition improves. Richardson[21] describes the treatment of two adult institutionalized patients with EEG-documented grand mal seizures, uncontrolled by medication, using this approach.

Relief (Avoidance) Program

Ounsted et al.[22] describe the relief (avoidance) technique in the case of a child with a documented spike and wave pattern on EEG. In this procedure an aversive stimulus such as photic stimulation during a spike-and-wave paroxysm appearing on an EEG record is administered. Administration of the noxious agent is continued until the subject demonstrates a reduction in either the clinical or electrical manifestations of the seizures.

Punishment Program

In the punishment program, a seizure is immediately followed by the administration of a noxious stimulus, such as an annoying electric shock, or a noise, or a flash of light. Efron[23] first described this technique in 1956. He was able in this way to train a patient to stop seizures once they had begun. Wright[24] presents another single case demonstrating use of this modality in a patient with documented neurogenic seizures, uncontrolled by medication.

Overt Reward Program

In the overt reward program, rewards are administered following totally seizure-free periods of time or following a particular time period during which there is a significant decrease in seizure rate. The criterion of a seizure-free time is gradually extended or the allowable number of seizures per unit time gradually reduced in an attempt to achieve full seizure control. Zlutnick et al.,[25] Sterman and Friar,[26] and Stevens[27] each cite instances of applying this strategy in patients with neurologically documented seizures, uncontrolled by medication.

Covert Reward Program

Daniels[28] has used a covert reward program in a case presumably of psychogenic origin (no EEG documentation). Seizure-provoking and non-seizure-provoking scenes are suggested to the patient while he or she is in a relaxed state. These scenes are immediately followed by imagined scenes of appropriate reward or non-reward as indicated. No tangible token, privilege, praise, or punishment is given; only the imagined representation is suggested to the patient.

Habituation or Extinction

Forster,[29] using classical conditioning techniques, has done much work in habituation training of various stimulus-evoked epilepsies. Where seizures are sensorily precipitated, this treatment strategy stipulates that the stimulus be presented below threshold and the intensity or frequency be gradually increased until the stimulus loses its seizure-evocative capacity. For example, repeated extinction trials were used to inhibit cortical hypersynchrony and clinical seizures in an adult patient who initially manifested paroxysmal EEG disturbances and photosensitive seizures during stroboscopic stimulation.[30]

Forster also successfully used extinction in other cases of photosensitive seizures.[31] Similarly, three patients with musicogenic epilepsy and anterior temporal EEG dysrhythmia[32] and one with reading-precipitated epilepsy[33] were also treated by extinction methods. Application of similar methods in a patient with somatosensory-evoked epilepsy and corresponding EEG abnormalities[34] as well as a patient with voice-induced epilepsy and associated temporal lobe EEG dysrhythmia[35] round out the list of seizure types so treated.

Conclusions

With the exception of Forster's work on habituation, frequently conducted with adult outpatients, conditioning strategies in the forms outlined above are most readily applied with children and with retarded patients in institutional settings. In these instances, the therapist has greater potential control over the contingencies of positive or negative reinforcement than with the more autonomously functioning patient. In the latter case the same principles of reward management may be applicable, but they may be operationally more effective if subtly integrated with a strategy for self-control, such as psychotherapy. In most instances, it requires a patient with greater ego strengths to successfully negotiate a strategy predicated on self-mastery.

PSYCHODYNAMIC APPROACHES

Psychodynamic approaches include psychotherapy and the identification of emotional triggers.

Psychoanalytically Oriented Psychotherapy

Gottschalk[36] describes how the seizure frequencies of three epileptic children, each with EEG documentation of diagnosis and each of whose seizures were not controlled by medication, decreased notably during and after a course of dynamically oriented psychotherapy consisting of at least one hundred individual sessions. The author cites evidence that both interpersonal events and intrapersonal conflicts activated epileptic behavior in these children. Elsewhere, Gottschalk[37] elaborates further on his thesis of the value of psychoanalytic psychotherapy in the management of certain types of epileptic patients.

Specific psychodynamic techniques are discussed in Part III of this book.

Identifying Emotional Triggers

Feldman and Paul[38] describe a technique of simulated recall and video replay which reduced seizure frequency in five patients with psychomotor epilepsy, documented by EEG and not controlled by medication. The authors contend that previous psychotherapeutic efforts had been unsuccessful because ictal amnesia had erased the memory of the stressful antecedent message-input which had triggered the seizures. Using videotaping of seizures and antecedent triggering events seemed helpful in enabling patients to either avoid or better cope with threatening environmental events.

Conclusions

The role of psychoanalytically oriented psychotherapy in the treatment of somatoform disorders and, hence, conversion seizures, is generally accepted.[39] What is not clear is why psychotherapy should be effective in the management of psychogenically precipitated neurogenic seizures. One plausible hypothesis may draw upon the frequently found suppression or limitation of paroxysmal activity during states of attention, stimulation, and concentration, particularly during periods of interest and high motivation.[40] A related postulate in this hypothesis is that these qualities of altered central nervous system arousal are part of the essential ingredients of any successful psychotherapeutic strategy and are indeed sustained in the patient if the psychotherapy is successful.[41] This theoretical frame of reference remains to be substantiated by further research.

RELAXATION AND HYPNOSIS

Relaxation techniques include relaxation, desensitization, and hypnosis.

Relaxation

All of the relaxation therapies share the features of muscular relaxation, regular practice, mental focusing, and task awareness.

Cabral and Scott[42] combined relaxation techniques with biofeedback (see below) to treat three patients with uncontrolled psychogenic seizures. The EEGs of two of the patients improved with both forms of treatment, while the EEG of the third improved only with biofeedback.

Desensitization

Parrino[43] describes the use of desensitization in an adult originally diagnosed as having Jacob-Creutzfeld Syndrome but subsequently found to have psychogenic seizures superimposed on a diffusely abnormal EEG. The patient was instructed to systematically relax and then think of a progressive hierarchy of anxiety-provoking scenes which had previously been established, by observation of the patient, to be seizure-provoking. Desensitization eventually achieved a seizure-free state.

Hypnosis

The role of hypnosis as an adjunctive aid in various somatoform disorders, including conversion seizures, is well documented.[44] Stein[45] reports the use of a technique entailing hypnotic relaxation and suggestion of a sense of mastery in treating one adolescent and two adults with EEG-documented seizure disorders uncontrolled by medication. Gardner[46] reports hypnotic treatment of an 8-year-old girl with EEG-documented familial epilepsy. Seizures uncontrolled by medication were thought to have a psychogenic component. A combination of play therapy, reinforcement, and hypnotherapy was used in the treatment. Williams et al.[47] report the treatment of three children and three adolescents by combining hypnosis with individual and family therapy as well as some behavior modification techniques for several types of uncontrolled seizures.

Conclusions

Reasoning by analogy may well be justified in this realm for heuristic purposes. Controlled studies of various relaxation therapies have shown each of them to be superior to placebo, and some to be superior to other techniques in treating certain psychophysiologic disorders. For example, in a review of various forms of relaxation therapy used as adjunctive aids in the clinical management of hypertension, Jacob et al.[48] found that superior and more sustained results were achieved by strategies employing various forms of relaxation therapy than by strategies employing only formal biofeedback procedures. Whether similar findings will be documented in the area of seizure disorders remains to be clarified by further research.

For best results, clinical experience suggests that relaxation techniques should be used in combination with other methods such as supportive psychotherapy.

BIOFEEDBACK

Biofeedback entails operant conditioning. The patient is instructed to generate or avoid generating a given bioelectric pattern or waveform. Correct or incorrect responses are appropriately fed back (for example, by visual or auditory signal) and may be actively rewarded or punished.

Sterman and coworkers[49] used sensorimotor rhythm (SMR) feedback training with four patients with EEG-documented seizures not controlled by anticonvulsant medications. Based on earlier experimental work with cats, this entailed positively reinforcing an EEG rhythm of 12 to 16 cycles per second (cps), which was found to inhibit seizures in the animals. The rate of seizures decreased; but the patients improved only as long as the biofeedback training sessions were continued. The authors themselves, however, note the possible role of nonspecific variables, reflecting the attention and concern shown to patients as distinct from the role of biofeedback.

Kaplan,[50] in a study of four patients with seizures uncontrolled by anticonvulsant medication, found that with biofeedback training significant improvement occurred in patients. However, since no significant EEG changes occurred which could be attributed to sensorimotor rhythm feedback training in these patients, the author postulates that nonspecific relaxation effects were responsible for the improvements noted. Gastaut[51] further emphasizes the need for caution in evaluating reports of presumed specificity of therapeutic effects of biofeedback in persons with epilepsy.

Responding to these concerns, Wyler et al.[52] conducted a study designed to rule out the placebo effect. They provided verbal and visual reinforcement to five patients under different sequences of two experimental conditions which were alternated over a 30-week period. These two conditions were: (a) when low voltage EEG fast activity over the frontal cortex was increased to an indicated criterion; or, (b) under a pseudo-conditioning paradigm in which reinforcement was given independent of EEG activity. Seizure frequency decreased significantly and specifically in condition (a) in two patients, attenuated under this condition in two others, and showed no change in one patient who was only given reinforcement for scalp EMG suppression.

Sterman and MacDonald[53] have also refuted a nonspecific interpretation of the effects of EEG biofeedback training. They studied the effects of such training in eight patients with poorly controlled seizures. Using a double or triple crossover design, training was based on simultaneous detection of two central cortical EEG frequency bands, with reward provided for the occurrence of one in the absence of the other. The design consisted of successive 3-month periods of training, with reward contingencies reversed after each period without the subject's knowledge. Six of the eight patients reported significant and sustained seizure reductions, which averaged 74 percent, following reward for either of the higher frequency bands (12-15 or 18-23 cps) in the absence of the lower frequency bands (6-9 cps). The authors advocate the concept of EEG "normalization" as a plausible explanation for the therapeutic effects of EEG feedback training.

Kuhlman,[54] in a similarly well-controlled evaluation of the effects of EEG feedback training, studied five patients with poorly controlled seizures.

During a 4- to 10-month period, he obtained quantitative analysis of seizures, the EEG, and serum anticonvulsant levels for each patient. Sustained seizure reduction did not occur during the first 4 to 5 weeks, in which feedback signals were presented randomly in relation to the EEG. However, when feedback was then made contingent upon central 9-14 cps activity, seizures declined by 60 percent in three patients. Power spectral analysis showed upward shifts in EEG frequency, decreases in abnormal slow activity, and enhancement of Alpha rhythm activity as a result of contingent training. Kuhlman concludes:

> 1. Significant seizure reductions can occur with EEG feedback training which are not related to placebo effects, non-specific factors or to changes in medication; 2. EEG changes associated with such training can best be described as "normalization"; 3. continued clinical investigation of EEG feedback training as a non-pharmacological adjunct to conventional therapy appears justified.

Yet Wyler and coworkers,[55] added a cautionary note in their subsequent report on the results of EEG feedback training with twenty-three severely epileptic patients. Their paradigm reinforced the patients' 18 Hz activity over the scalp approximation of their focus while suppressing temporalis EMG and low frequency EEG activity. In contrast to other studies using EEG feedback, only 43 percent of patients showed significant changes in seizure occurrence and a lesser number were felt to have benefitted clinically. Although a few patients were substantially helped by their training, the mechanism for this effect was noted to be unclear.

DISCUSSION OF SPECIALIZED TREATMENT TECHNIQUES

The preceding discussion of treatment techniques indicates the multiplicity of approaches that have been used as adjuncts in the management of uncontrolled seizure disorders. These various techniques are not mutually exclusive; in fact, they are often combined in practice. They may, indeed, share common features—such as progressive relaxation, attention activation, generation of positive expectancies, implicit or explicit reward/punishment features, and emotional support—that are more uniformly operative in each than the proponents of the different methodologies might readily acknowledge. As a group, the reports of these treatments call attention to the importance of environmental, interpersonal, and intrapsychic factors in influencing seizure frequency in many patients. Indeed, in some of the reports cited, not only was improved seizure control achieved by the stated intervention, but this improvement was also maintained to a degree allowing substantial reduction of anticonvulsant doses, with consequent diminution of associated side effects.

Of the treatment techniques discussed, the recent studies in EEG feedback training have the advantage of most methodological precision, controlled experimental design, and hence greatest demonstrated specificity in ruling out placebo effects. However, these advantages are somewhat offset at present by the rather elaborate and expensive technology required for effective EEG feedback training and monitoring, which limits its availability. If the favorable results of some workers in this area continue to be sustained by further studies, it seems probable that advances in miniaturization and mass production of training and monitoring components could readily enhance their availability.

An alternate or complementary consideration might entail exploring the psychological correlates of EEG "normalization." This could involve EEG-monitored studies of the purported process of "normalized" central nervous system arousal, which has been posited as the mechanism of efficacy of the conditioning, psychotherapy and relaxation strategies previously outlined above. Or, from another perspective, it could involve careful psychometric assessment of the emotional and cognitive correlates of EEG feedback training, which has not been done in detail to date. It is of interest that Cobb,[56] using eclectically based psychiatric treatment of carefully selected drug-resistant seizure patients in the days antedating biofeedback availability, obtained results similar to those of the best current biofeedback workers, in terms of percentage of favorable clinical responders (67 percent showed marked improvement and 10 percent slight improvement). Whether similar evidence of generalizability across treatment techniques will be documented in the area of seizure disorders remains to be clarified by further research.

Finally, just as no single medication has emerged that is uniformly efficacious for all seizure patients, so also is no single psychotherapeutic or psychobiological modality uniformly effective in the cases uncontrolled by anticonvulsant medication. As the neurologist may need to go through multiple clinical trials in attempting to formulate an anticonvulsant regimen best suited to the patient's need, so must the mental health practitioner be prepared to reformulate his or her treatment strategy based on the patient's pattern of response. It follows logically that it behooves the practitioner to have a diversified therapeutic armamentarium available to this end.

The Neurologist and
the Mental Health Practitioner

The desirability of a close working relationship with the neurologist cannot be overemphasized. Such an effective combined approach can help forestall the frequent tendency toward unwarranted, dichotomous thinking on the part of the patient and others as to whether the problem is either "purely" neurological or "purely" psychological. It has been noted[57] that often the neurologist and the mental health practitioner themselves are unsure about the relative contributions of neurogenic and psychogenic factors in cases of uncontrolled seizures. In such instances, the capacity to work in a complementary fashion on both of these fronts is both clinically sound and reassuring to the patient.

The importance of combining the special techniques centered on seizure control with an overall psychotherapeutic strategy to meet the ongoing needs of the patient with epilepsy should be noted. Of necessity, a thorough assessment of various possible sources of stress contributing to uncontrolled seizures will have been part of the clinician's formulation of an effective treatment strategy to bring the seizures under improved control. A reasonable extension of this process will be advising the patient and his or her family about continuing strategies to either diminish unwarranted stress or to enhance the patient's capacities for coping with that stress which is unavoidable.

REFERENCES

1. Commission for the Control of Epilepsy and its Consequences. *Plan for Nationwide Action on Epilepsy.* U.S. Dept. of HEW, National Institutes of Health, Bethesda, Vol. II, Part 2, 1977, p. 393-402; Minter, R. E. Can emotions precipitate seizures—A review of the question. *Journal of Family Practice.* 8:55-59, 1979.
2. Groethuysen, U.C., Robinson, D. B., Haylett, C. H., et al. Depth electrographic recording of a seizure during a structured interview. *Psychosomat. Med.*, 19:353-632, 1957. Stevens, J. R. Central and peripheral factors in epileptic discharge. *Arch. Neurol.*, 7:330-338, 1962. Small, J. G., Stevens, J. R., Milstein, V. Electroclinical correlates of emotional activation of the electroencephalogram. *J. Nerv. Ment. Dis.*, 138:146-155, 1964.
3. Allen, I. M. The emotional factor and the epileptic attack. *N.Z. Med. J.*, 55:297, 1956.
4. Mignone, R. J., Donnelly, E. F., Sadowsky, O. Psychological and neurological comparisons of psychomotor and non-psychomotor epileptic patients. *Epilepsia*, 11:345, 1970.
5. Swinyard, E. A., Miyahara, J. T., Clark, L. D., et al. The effect of experimentally-induced stress on pentylenetetrazol threshold in mice. *Psychopharmacologia*, 4:343-353, 1963.
6. Martinek, Z., and Horak, F. Development of so called "genuine" epileptic seizures in dogs during emotional excitement. *Physiol. Bohemoslov.*, 19:185-195, 1970.
7. Kopeloff, L. M., Chusid, J. G., Kopeloff, N. Chronic experimental epilepsy in Macaca mulatta. *Neurology*, 4:218-227, 1954. Lockard, J. S., Wilson, W. L., Uhlir, V. Spontaneous seizure frequency and avoidance conditioning in monkeys. *Epilepsia*, 13:437-444, 1972.
8. Glaser, G. Convulsive Disorders. In: H. Merritt (ed.) *Textbook of Neurology*, 6th Ed. Lea & Febiger, Philadelphia, 1979, p. 813-882; Mostofsky, D. I. and Balaschak, B. Psychobiological control of seizures, *Psychol. Bull.* 84:723-750, 1977. Williams, D. T., Spiegel, H., Mostofsky, D. I. Neurogenic and hysterical seizures in children and adolescents: differential diagnostic and therapeutic considerations. *Am. J. Psychiatry*, 135:82-86, 1978.
9. Task Force on Nomenclature and Statistics of the American Psychiatric Association. *Diagnostic and Statistical Manual of Mental Disorders, Third Edition*, American Psychiatric Association, Washington, D.C., 1980.
10. Desai, B. T., Riley, T. L., Porter, R. J., et al. Active noncompliance as a cause of uncon-

trolled seizures. *Epilepsia*, 19:447-452, 1978.

11. Solomon, G., and Plum, F. *Clinical management of seizures*. Philadelphia: W. B. Saunders Co., 1976.

12. Peterson, D. B., Sumner, J. N. and Jones, G. A. Role of hypnosis in differentiation of epileptic from convulsive-like seizures. *Am. J. Psychiatry*, 107:438-432, 1950. Sumner, J. W., Rameron, R. R., and Peterson, D. B. Hypnosis in differentiation of epileptic from convulsive-like seizures. *Neurology*, 2:395-402, 1952. Schwarz, B. E., Bickford, R. G., and Rasmussen, W. C. Hypnotic phenomena, including hypnotically activated seizures, studies with the EEG. *J. Nerv. Ment. Dis.*, 122:564-574, 1955.

13. Ramani, S. V., Quesney, L. F., Olson, D. et al. Diagnosis of hysterical seizures in epileptic patients. *Am. J. Psychiatry*, 137:705-709, 1980.

14. Williams, D. T., Gold, A. P., Shrout, P., et al. The impact of psychiatric intervention on patients with uncontrolled seizures. *J. Nerv. Ment. Dis.*, 167:626-631, 1979.

15. Remick, R. A., and Wada, J. A. Complex partial and pseudoseizure disorders. *Am. J. Psychiatry*, 136:320-323, 1979.

16. Rossen, R. EEG studies in idiopathic epilepsy and syncope. *Am. J. Psychiatry*, 104:391, 1947.

17. Peterson, D. B., Sumner, J. N. and Jones, G. A. Role of hypnosis in differentiation of epileptic from convulsive-like seizures. *Am. J. Psychiatry*, 107:428-432, 1950. Sumner, J. W., Rameron, R. R., and Peterson, D. B. Hypnosis in differentiation of epileptic from convulsive-like seizures. *Neurology*, 2:395-402, 1952.

18. Ives, J. and Wood, J. 4-Channel 24 hour cassette recorder for longterm EEG monitoring of ambulatory patients. *Electroenceph. Clin. Neurophysiol.* 39:88-92, 1975.

19. Mostofsky, E. I. and Balaschak, B. Psychobiological control of seizures. *Psychol. Bull.* 84:723-750, 1977.

20. Gardner, J. Behavior therapy treatment approach to a psychogenic seizure case. *J. Consult. Psychol.*, 31:209-212, 1967.

21. Richardson, R. Environmental contingencies in seizure disorders. Presented at *Assoc. for Advancement of Behav. Ther.*, New York, 1972.

22. Ounsted, C., Lee, D., and Hutt, S. J. Electroencephalographic and clinical changes in an epileptic child during repeated photic stimulation. *Electroenceph. & Clin. Neurophysiol.*, 21:388-391, 1966.

23. Efron, R. The effect of olfactory stimuli in arresting uncinate fits. *Brain*, 79:267-281, 1956. Efron, R. The conditioned inhibition of uncinate fits. *Brain*, 80:251-262, 1957.

24. Wright, L. Aversive conditioning of self-induced seizures. *Behavior Therapy*. 4:712-713, 1973.

25. Zlutnick, S., et al. Behavioral control of seizure disorders. In: R. Katz and S. Zlutnick (eds.) *Behavior Therapy and Health Care: Principles and Applications*. New York: Pergamon Press, 1975.

26. Sterman, M. and Friar, L. Suppression of seizures in an epileptic following sensorimotor EEG feedback training. *Electroenceph. & Clin. Neurophysiol.* 33:89-95, 1972.

27. Stevens, J. Endogenous conditioning to abnormal cerebral electrical transients in man. *Science*, 137:974-976, 1962.

28. Daniels, L. The treatment of grand mal epilepsy by covert and operant conditioning techniques: a case study. *Psychosomatic Medicine.* 16:65-67, 1975.

29. Forster, F. The classification and conditioning of the reflex epilepsies. *Intl. J. Neurology.* 9:73-86, 1972.

30. Forster, F. and Campos, G. Conditioning factors in stroboscopic and induced seizures. *Epilepsia.* 5:156-165, 1964.

31. Forster, F., et al. Stroboscopic-induced seizure discharges: modification by extinction techniques. *Arch. Neurol.*, 11:603-608, 1964. Forster, F., et al. Auditory clicks in extinction of stroboscope-induced seizures. *Epilepsia*, 6:217-225, 1965. Forster, F., et al. Computer automation of the conditioning therapy of stroboscopic induced seizures. *Transact. Am. Neurol. Assoc.*, pp. 232-233, 1966.

32. Forster, F., et al. Conditioning in musicogenic epilepsy. *Transact. Am. Neurol. Assoc.*, pp. 236-237, 1967.

33. Forster, F., et al. Clinical therapeutic conditioning in reading epilepsy. *Neurology*, 19:717-723, 1969.
34. Forster, F. and Cleeland, C. Somatosensory evoked epilepsy. *Transact. Am. Neurol. Assoc.* 94:268-269, 1969.
35. Forster, F., et al. A case of voice-induced epilepsy treated by conditioning. *Neurology*, 19:319-325, 1969.
36. Gottschalk, L. Effects of intensive psychotherapy on epileptic children. *Arch. Neurol. & Psychiat.*, 70:361-384, 1953.
37. Gottschalk, L. A. The relationship of psychologic state and epileptic activity: psychoanalytic observations on an epileptic child. *The Psychoanalytic Study of the Child*. New Haven: Yale University Press, 1956.
38. Feldman, R. and Paul, N. Identity of emotional triggers in epilepsy. *J. Nerv. & Ment. Dis.*, 1962:343-353, 1976.
39. Nemiah, J. C. Hysterical neurosis, conversion type. In: A. Freedman, H. Kaplan and B. Sadock (eds.), *Comprehensive Textbook of Psychiatry*, 2nd Ed., Baltimore, MD: Williams & Wilkins, 1975.
40. Glaser, G. Epilepsy—neuropsychological aspects. In: M. Reiser (ed.), *American Handbook of Psychiatry*, Vol. IV, New York: Basic Books, 1975, p. 314-355.
41. Frank, J. D., Hoehn-Saric, R., Imber, S. D., et al. *Effective Ingredients of Successful Psychotherapy*. New York: Brunner/Mazel, 1978.
42. Cabral, R. J. and Scott, D. S. The effects of desensitization techniques, biofeedback and relaxation on intractable epilepsy. *J. Neurol. Neurosurg. Psychiatry*, 39:504-507, 1976.
43. Parrino, J. Reduction of seizures by desensitization. *J. Behav. Ther. & Exp. Psychiat.*, 2:215-218, 1971.
44. Spiegel, H., & Spiegel, D. *Trance and Treatment: Clinical Uses of Hypnosis*. New York: Basic Books, 1978. Williams, D. and Singh, M. Hypnosis as a facilitating therapeutic adjunct in child psychiatry. *J. Am. Acad. Ch. Psychiat.*, 15:326-342, 1976.
45. Stein, C. The clenched fist technique as a hypnotic procedure in clinical psychotherapy, *Am. J. Clin. Hypn.*, 6:113-119, 1963.
46. Gardner, G. Use of hypnosis for psychogenic epilepsy in a child. *Am. J. Clin. Hypn.*, 15:166-169, 1973.
47. Williams, D. T., Spiegel, H., and Mostofsky, D. I. Neurogenic and hysterical seizures in children and adolescents: differential diagnostic and therapeutic considerations. *Am. J. Psychiatry*, 135:82-86, 1978.
48. Jacob, R. G., Kraemer, H. C., and Agras, W. S. Relaxation therapy in the treatment of hypertension. *Arch. Gen. Psychiatry*, 34:1417-1427, 1977.
49. Sterman, M. Neurophysiologic and clinical studies of sensorimotor EEG biofeedback training: some effects on epilepsy. *Seminars in Psychiat.*, 5:507-525, 1973. Sterman, M., et al. Biofeedback training of the sensorimotor EEG rhythm in man: Effects on epilepsy. *Epilepsia*, 15:395-416, 1974.
50. Kaplan, B. Biofeedback in epileptics: Equivocal relationship of reinforced EEG frequency to seizure reduction. *Epilepsia*, 16:477-485, 1975.
51. Gastaut, H. Comments on biofeedback in epileptics. *Epilepsia*, 16:487-490, 1975.
52. Wyler, A. R., Lockard, J. S., Ward, A. A., et al., Conditioned EEG desynchronization and seizure occurrence in patients. *Electroenceph. Clin. Neurophysiol.*, 41:501-512, 1976.
53. Sterman, M. B. and MacDonald, L. R. Effects of central cortical EEG feedback training on incidence of poorly controlled seizures. *Epilepsia*, 19:207-22, 1978.
54. Kuhlman, W. N. EEG feedback training of epileptic patients: clinical and electroencephalographic analysis. *Electroenceph. Clin. Neurophysiol.*, 45:699-710, 1978.
55. Wyler, A. R., Robbins, C. A., and Dodrill, C. B. EEG operant conditioning for control of epilepsy. *Epilepsia*, 20:279-286, 1979.
56. Cobb, S. Psychiatric approach to the treatment of epilepsy. *Am. J. Psychiatry*, 96:1009, 1940.
57. Williams, D. T., Gold, A. P., Shrout, P., et al., The impact of psychiatric intervention on patients with uncontrolled seizures. *J. Nerv. Ment. Dis.*, 167:626-631, 1979.

II.
INFORMATION FOR PSYCHOSOCIAL ASSESSMENT

3

NEUROBIOLOGICAL BASIS OF PSYCHOPATHOLOGY ASSOCIATED WITH EPILEPSY

IRA SHERWIN, M.D.

Although none would deny that the brain is the organ of the mind, any attempt to define the specific relationships between selected mental activities and restricted neuronal assemblies immediately leads us into the realm of controversy. This stems, in part, from the fact that the doctrine of cerebral localization is often misconstrued to mean that specific mental functions reside in restricted neural ensembles. This is almost certainly incorrect. It is correct, however, to claim that damage restricted to certain localized brain regions may produce highly specific disturbances in mental activities.

For example, although it would be incorrect to argue that language function resides in Broca's and Wernicke's areas of the left hemisphere, it is abundantly clear that small lesions in these areas produce aphasias while similar lesions in the right hemisphere do not. Analogously, although small lesions in many brain regions have little or no effect on consciousness, comparable lesions in the reticular formation selectively produce marked alterations of consciousness. Other examples would include the selective disturbance of recent memory seen in Korsakoff's disease, resulting, most likely, from damage to the hippocampal-mamillary body circuit. The most parsimonious explanation for the specificity of these relationships is that certain specific mental functions are critically dependent upon the integrity of certain restricted brain regions. It is when these regions are damaged that the disturbances of specific mental activities become manifest. It should be appreciated that this concept is vastly different from that of neural centers, that is, that specific mental functions reside in specific brain regions.

This work was supported by the Veterans Administration and the USPHS (Grant #NS02808).

Perhaps the most striking of these relationships, and the one of principal concern to us, is the association of epileptic lesions—particularly limbic, that is, temporal lobe epileptic lesions—and disturbances of behavior. This tendency for psychopathology to develop in association with epilepsy has been recognized since ancient times.[1] It may not be unduly extravagant to say that in no other disorder do the disciplines of neurology and psychiatry overlap so extensively as in epilepsy. In more recent times, however, partly as a result of having demonstrated disordered cerebral electrogenesis in epileptic patients and partly as a result of well-intentioned efforts to destigmatize epilepsy, a continuing effort began seeking to repudiate and deny the notion of this association.[2,3] This is exemplified by the current pronouncement of the professional advisory board of the Epilepsy Foundation of America:

> Since personality is regarded as a socially-acquired characteristic, there is no convincing evidence suggesting any particular set of behavioral attitudes or disorder resulting directly from seizures. However, the fact of epilepsy may have considerable impact on the individual's social experiences. The persons with epilepsy may encounter very similar social situations—overprotectiveness or a wide swing in emotional reactions on the part of parents, ostracism or taunting from peers—which have damaging effects on personality whether epilepsy is present or not. The child who faces these social and family problems compensates by fighting back. Thus, while some persons with epilepsy may display behavioral problems, it should be remembered that these may be normal reactions to abnormal situations.[4]

As a consequence, many of the serious psychiatric complications of epilepsy have often gone unrecognized by the internist or neurologist and by and large have been of little interest to the psychiatrist. The result has been that many epilepsy patients continue to receive only incomplete treatment for a serious and complex problem. The true extent of this problem is difficult to estimate. Recently the Commission for the Control of Epilepsy and Its Consequences reported that "12% of the 200,000 persons in institutions for the mentally ill have epilepsy."[5] This is a remarkable finding in itself, because it is commonly estimated that the prevalence of epilepsy in the general population is only about 1 percent. Additionally, however, when it is realized that these hospitalized patients represent only the most serious cases, it is probable that in terms of the actual prevalence of psychopathology associated with epilepsy this statistic is extremely conservative.

In this chapter, the various facets of this relationship will be explored in detail. I shall attempt to show that there exists not only a generally increased prevalence of psychopathology in association with epilepsy, but that there is a high degree of specificity between the type of epilepsy and the type of associated psychopathology. It is only through an increased awareness of the details of these associations that the physician can begin to provide patients with this syndrome the comprehensive care they require.

THE "EPILEPTIC PERSONALITY"

Many and varied psychopathological features have been described in persons with epilepsy. Nosologically these range from character disorders to psychosis. In considering the complex nature of the relationships between the epilepsies and the various types of associated psychopathology, it is useful to distinguish the transient peri-ictal (near the time of a seizure) psychiatric features from the persistent inter-ictal (between seizure) psychopathological states. Numerous case reports indicate that psychiatric abnormalities may occur as peri-ictal phenomena. For the most part, however, the inter-ictal psychopathies appear to predominate.

Certain features have been considered to constitute an "epileptic personality." Although reports vary, several personality traits form a common thread running across and binding together these descriptions. The essential features include a day-to-day variability and unpredictability of behavior, characterized by irritability, and an explosive temperament that alternates with an unctuous good-naturedness. There is a deepening of emotional responsiveness and heightening of egocentricity characterized by "oceanic ideation" and religious fervor. There is an excessive concern with seemingly trivial events, characterized by verboseness in speaking and writing. Clinically, the perseverative and circumstantial nature of these productions is appreciated as a "sticky or adhesive" quality. Beyond these peculiarities of personality, many studies indicate that a detailed psychological evaluation of the epileptic patient frequently reveals more serious forms of psychopathology.

BEHAVIOR AND EPILEPSY TYPE

Some authors, although acknowledging a special association between psychopathology and epilepsy, view this as an indirect association. For example, the psychiatric features seen in persons with epilepsy are often considered to be a consequence of problems in social adaptation that stem from having a disease which stigmatizes and which frequently results in discrimination and ostracism. Admittedly, such social factors may aggravate the problems of psychological adjustment faced by epilepsy patients. However, in themselves they cannot account for certain characteristic psychopathological entities (for example, the schizophrenic-like psychosis) repeatedly noted in epileptics. Other stigmatizing chronic diseases, for example tuberculosis, have not been associated with the distinctive psychopathological features specifically attributed to persons with epilepsy.[6] Chronic treatment with anticonvulsants has, in an analogous manner, been implicated by some as being causative of the increased prevalence of psychiatric disorders in epilepsy patients.[7] Although it is well established that both acute and chronic psychiatric syndromes may occur as toxic manifestations of anticonvulsant therapy, it appears most unlikely that this can account for the bulk of the psychiatric features occurring in epilepsy patients. This view gains support from the fact that well before the introduction of anticonvulsants numerous reports appeared describing psychopathological features occurring in association with epilepsy[8,9,10] that differ little from those accounts which followed the introduction of these therapeutic agents.

In part, too, these discrepant views stem from a failure to make distinctions between the various types of epilepsy, when considering "associated" disorders of behavior. With the advent of modern electroencephalographic (EEG) technology,[11] a special association of severe psychiatric disorders with the psychomotor (temporal lobe) form of epilepsy was documented. Interest in this association of epilepsy—in particular, temporal lobe epilepsy (TLE)—with various forms of behavioral disorder has produced a rich but confusing and often contradictory literature. This is due in part to the loose nosology characterizing much of the psychiatric literature and in part to the varying neurological and EEG criteria chosen for making the diagnosis of TLE. Diagnostic difficulties arise on the one hand from the protean manifestations which characterize the clinical seizures and on the other from the fact that electrical discharges deep in the temporal lobe frequently go undetected in the scalp-recorded EEG.

On balance, however, current evidence suggests that Gibbs's statement that the Sylvian fissure divides neurology from psychiatry[12] was not unreasonable. By this he meant that patients with epileptogenic foci above the Sylvian fissure tend to present to neurologists, while those with foci below the fissure present to psychiatrists.

For our purposes, the individual temporal lobe seizures of TLE may be defined operationally as "focal seizures produced by discharging lesions situated in or (secondarily) projecting to the temporal lobes."[13] It would undoubtedly be more correct to speak of limbic rather than temporal lobe epilepsy, since many clinical features appear to depend upon the propagation of the discharges from the temporal lobe per se into structures with which the temporal lobes have major anatomical connections, for example, the hypothalamus. However, because the appellation TLE is so widely used, we shall follow this terminology. At present, the diagnosis of TLE depends primarily upon the symptomatology of the clinical seizures. This situation may soon change due to a new radiographic technique, Positron Emission Tomography, which promises to be most useful in detecting deeply placed electrically silent (by EEG) epileptogenic foci. The technique depends upon the selective uptake of a radio-fluorine tagged form of glucose by metabolically active brain sites.

In focal epilepsy other than TLE, the seizures are characterized by elementary neurological signs and symptoms (paresthesias, myoclonic movements, etc.). Temporal lobe seizures often share some features in common with other types of focal and/or generalized seizures. In the main, however, they tend to be characterized by complex sensory, motor, and autonomic disturbances superimposed on a background of altered consciousness. The most characteristic seizures seen in psychomotor (temporal lobe) epilepsy are automatisms. These include chewing, licking and smacking of the lips, and a variety of inappropriate but purposeful movements. The various signs and symptoms characterizing these seizures may be grouped into four major categories: somatomotor, sensory, psychical, and autonomic phenomena. For additional details of the neurological manifestations, see Chapter 1.

For our purposes, the psychical phenomena require special consideration. Since Gibbs' original suggestion equating psychomotor *seizures* with temporal lobe *epilepsy*,[14] it has become increasingly clear that patients with epilepsy arising from brain sites other than the temporal lobes may also have complex partial (psychomotor) seizures. It is also now well known that temporal lobe epilepsy patients may have generalized seizures either as their only ictal manifestation or in combination with complex partial seizures. Because different types of epilepsy may have certain seizure patterns in common, it becomes exceedingly difficult to evaluate the relative prevalence of the psychopathology described in those studies that compare "grand-mal epileptics" with "psychomotor epileptics" or with "temporal lobe epileptics." This is especially so when the diagnosis of the type of epilepsy is based primarily on the symptomatology of the seizures. These difficulties notwithstanding, the principle that certain specific types of epilepsy are more likely to be associated with some forms of psychopathy than are other types is strongly supported by the fact that this association is rarely encountered in patients with Bravais-Jacksonian Epilepsy.[15]

DISORDERS OF BEHAVIOR DURING SEIZURES

Psychopathological states that occur as ictal or peri-ictal events, although they are unquestionably related to the patient's epilepsy in a highly specific manner, are, in fact, rare phenomena.

Hallucinations

Among the various ictal psychical phenomena that occur in TLE, hallucinatory experiences are common. The most characteristic and well known of these is the so-called olfactory hallucination or uncinate fit. The hallucinated odor typically has an unpleasant (stenchlike) quality often described as disgusting and rarely, if ever, as pleasant.[16] Formed visual hallucinations may occur and are more common when the epileptogenic focus is in the right temporal lobe.

Ictal Disturbances of Consciousness

The reticular formation, a system of nerve fibers and cells occupying the medial portion of the brain stem from the medulla to the thalamus, plays a major role in consciousness, wakefulness, and attention. Seizures either arising in or propagating to the reticular formation may produce unconsciousness. Of perhaps more interest are the altered states of consciousness that may occur as part of a seizure; and of still greater interest are those disorders of consciousness that are the sole manifestation of a seizure. In the latter states, the patient is not unconscious; rather, the patient is unaware of his or her surroundings and may behave in an inappropriate, albeit purposeful, manner. The "dreamy-state" described by Hughlings Jackson is a classical example of this. A key feature central to these states is an impairment in the ability to lay down new memory traces.

Ictal Amnesia

The critical role played by the medial temporal structures in elaborating recent memory has been thoroughly documented.[17,18,19] Seizures arising in these structures may be characterized by an ictal amnesia. Their shorter duration and the lack of hypermnesia for the beginning and end of the amnesic period distinguish such fits from fugue states. One highly characteristic ictal memory disturbance in TLE is that of *déja vu* and, less commonly, *jamais vu*. These misperceptions of familiarity and unfamiliarity occur more frequently when the epileptogenic focus involves the right temporal lobe.[20] Patients with TLE may also complain of poor memory (inter-ictal amnesia) which, in practice, is usually difficult to document. It may be that this is actually a result of the fact that *memorizing* becomes defective during periods of repeated subclinical seizures—that this is an ictal memory disturbance. Related to ictal disorders of memory is *forced thinking*. In this type of seizure, consciousness is suddenly interrupted by the feeling of a forced channeling of the patient's thoughts.

Ictal Disturbances of Sexuality

Sexual disorders have repeatedly been reported to occur in association with epilepsy. Because of the very important role played by the limbic system in sexual behavior, it is not too surprising that limbic (temporal lobe) epilepsy in particular is often associated with sexual dysfunction. The possibility that there might be a common functional substrate shared by the mechanisms subserving sexual function and epileptic seizures has been recognized since antiquity.[21] Through the ensuing years, many aspects of sexuality have been related to epilepsy in a variety of more or less specific ways. Only relatively recently, largely due to studies using modern electrophysiological techniques, have the complex interrelationships between sexuality and epilepsy become separable from the myths surrounding them. In analyzing these relationships, we will first consider the ictal disorders of sexuality; inter-ictal disorders are discussed on pages 87-89.

The term *ictal disturbances of sexuality* is used to refer to instances in which some clinical manifestations of the seizure are sexual in nature. It is probably more correct to speak of peri-ictal disturbances of sexuality, since certain sexual features occur in the immediate pre- and post-ictal periods. Such disturbances in sexuality fall into two main categories. In the first, and more common, the seizure occurs in the absence of any obvious precipitating event and may be characterized by frank sexual behavior (motor activity) or experience (sensory seizures). In the second category, sexual activity may precipitate a seizure that may or may not have some sexual features. This is a special form of the more general type of seizure disorder, often termed *reflex epilepsy*.

Public Undressing. An example of the seizure characterized by sexual behavior is the automatism in which disrobing in public may occur, either as part of a seizure or in the confusional state that characterizes the immediate post-ictal period. When ictal disrobing occurs as the sole manifestation of a seizure disorder, the psychiatric diagnosis of exhibitionism is often made.[22] Clinical features that should arouse the suspicion of epilepsy in supposed cases of exhibitionism are: other manifestations suggestive of a seizure disorder; its occurrence in females; and the fact that in true exhibitionism the display is usually made in view of a specifically selected victim, whereas in epilepsy the display is made indiscriminately. These features are of only limited value for differential diagnosis, and a thorough neurological workup is indicated.

Genital Paresthesias. Seizures characterized by genital paresthesias and erotic sensations have been reported by several authors,[23,24] most of whose patients were shown to have temporal lobe epilepsy.

Erotomania and Nymphomania. One other type of seizure in this category that deserves special comment is exemplified by the case of erotomania (nymphomania) reported by Erickson.[25] The patient's attacks were characterized by "a hot feeling all over, as if she were having intercourse." Subsequently these hot spells became associated with jerking movements of the left arm and leg. Following the onset of a left hemiparesis, the patient underwent craniotomy, with the removal of a right rolandic parasaggital hemangioma. After this the "passionate spells" ceased, and the patient retained what she called "normal sexual desire."

The location of this tumor in the parasaggital portion of the frontal lobe, that is, the region for the cortical representation of the genitalia, probably accounts for the ictal genital paresthesias. That frontal lobe dysfunction might be the most likely cause of the patient's erotomania is in keeping with the observation that most other instances of erotomania secondary to organic brain disease occur in cases of dementia paralytica and senile dementia, disorders that involve the frontal lobes.[26] The most probable mechanism involved is a loss of the normal inhibition exerted on the limbic system by the frontal lobes. Thus it seems that in this case the ictal events, that is, focal (genital) sensory seizures in the presence of frontal lobe dysfunction, were interpreted as sexual arousal (erotomania). Additionally, the patient had an inter-ictal sexual disorder (nymphomania) probably reflecting the release of limbic activity secondary to the frontal lobe dysfunction.

Mixed Reflex and Nonreflex Epilepsy. Recently Bancaud et al.[27] described a case that shares features in common with this group of ictal sexual disorders and also with the other main group of ictal sexual disorders, that is, the reflex epilepsies. A young woman whose seizures were ushered in by a feeling of fear would then lift her skirts in public and rub herself with a closed fist. Over time, the sensation of fear was replaced by a pleasurable feeling similar to that which she experienced during masturbation. Subsequently, the seizures became reflex in character in that she would deliberately induce similar attacks by masturbating. At surgery, an astrocytoma was found involving the right amygdala and hippocampus.

Reflex Epilepsy. In contrast to the mixed case described above, Hoenig and Hamilton[28] reported what appears to be an unequivocal case of "reflex sexual epilepsy." In reflex epilepsy with a sexual component, the seizures themselves are not sexual in character but rather are triggered by a specific sexual act, in this case orgasm. Hoenig and Hamilton's patient, a 32-year-old married woman, complained of spells immediately following orgasm. The spells were characterized by pallor, loss of consciousness, and twitching of the left arm and leg. Seizures did not occur on those rare occasions when intercourse was not accompanied by orgasm, suggesting that the critical trigger was the orgasm per se, and not peripheral tactile stimulation. Treatment with anticonvulsants markedly reduced the number of attacks.

Frequency of Occurrence. The neurophysiological substrate involved in these curious seizures is considered later, in the section on inter-ictal sexual disturbances. For now it is important to stress the fact that, although more dramatic, these ictal disturbances are much less common than the inter-ictal disorders of sexuality.

Ictal Emotion

Various feeling states (emotions) may occur as ictal events. An often cited example is the state of ecstasy described by Dostoevski as a part of his seizures. More frequent, however, is a sensation of fear or dread, which seems to occur most often with amygdala seizures. A curious and often embarrassing ictal emotional disturbance characterizes gelastic epilepsy. The unbidden bursts of laughter are most frequently associated with temporal lobe epilepsy, although a hypothalamic origin has been presumed in some cases.

Ictal Aggression

Of special interest are those aggressive acts in persons with epilepsy which occur as part of an ictal episode. These are of particular concern not only because of what they might reveal about the neuroanatomical substrates of emotion and behavior but because of their medico-legal significance. The older epilepsy literature refers to a clinical state called "epileptic mania." The term was used to describe senseless destructive acts in patients who, in addition, had typical convulsive seizures.

A special form of such peri-ictal aggressiveness was described by Meyer.[29] He termed it "mania transitoria." By this he meant that the aggressive, destructive act was the sole ictal manifestation. In recent years, this notion has been resurrected under the ambiguous rubric of the "episodic dyscontrol syndrome."[30] In a recent paper purporting to define the "Neurology of Explosive Rage," F. A. Elliot states, "The term 'dyscontrol syndrome' is sometimes used for symptoms arising from poor impulse control, whether the cause is organic or functional. It is an important cause of wife and child battery, senseless assaults, motiveless homicides, self-injury, dangerously aggressive driving, domestic infelicity, divorce and (in children) educational difficulties."[31] Apparently the only calamities to befall mankind for which this is not an "important cause" are acts of God!

For those cases where there is no apparent cause, the notion of an "epileptoid-mechanism" has been contrived to account for the episodic dyscontrol syndrome. That episodic dyscontrol seductively invites comparison with the paroxysmal nature of epileptic seizures is understandable. However, the introduction of the term "epileptoid" is tautological and leads to such self-fulfilling prophecies as "the concept of episodic dyscontrol with an 'epileptoid' mechanism could be established on the basis of a careful phenomenologic analysis of behavior."[32] It would seem that if the cause of the dyscontrol syndrome is in reality epilepsy, then nothing is gained by substituting the word "epileptoid." If, as it appears, the only relationship of the dyscontrol syndrome to epilepsy is the absence of a demonstrable cause (including epilepsy), then the use of the term "epileptoid" is at best an obfuscation and at worst impedes the analysis of those disorders of behavior which are truly related to epilepsy.

The legitimacy of this notion aside, such an entity is frequently invoked as a legal defense. Yet, based on his personal experience with a series of one thousand court reports, MacDonald was able to find "only two examples of crimes committed as a result of an epileptic seizure."[33] Knox, in a review of the records of 434 unselected epileptics attending a single clinic, was able to find only one case in which peri-ictal aggressiveness was a clinical feature.[34] Gunn and Fenton, in a complementary study, analyzed the histories of 32 epileptic patients who were committed because of crimes of violence. More than half of these patients were found to be cases of TLE. In only two patients, however, were there aggressive acts that appeared to occur peri-ictally. In both cases the aggressive acts appeared to be a part of the immediate post-ictal confusional state.[35]

It appears from the foregoing that although aggressive behavior is an infrequent ictal or peri-ictal phenomenon in epilepsy patients in general, it may occur specifically in a small but important number of cases of TLE. Despite this, it must be stressed that aggressivity as the sole ictal manifestation in epilepsy of any type must be exceedingly rare, if, in fact, it ever occurs. As an inter-ictal phenomenon, aggressivity appears to be common and will be considered in detail below.

DISORDERS OF BEHAVIOR BETWEEN SEIZURES

The "epileptic personality" described on page 79 is the most frequently cited inter-ictal behavior disorder. A commonly noted feature in this disorder is an irritable temperament often expressed in acts of aggression.

Inter-ictal Aggressivity

Unlike the acts of aggression seen in psychopathic patients, the aggressive behavior in epilepsy patients does not constitute a life-style. It must be stressed that this does not imply that the aggressive acts appear de novo in a paroxysmal fashion. In point of fact, there is often an identifiable precipitant. Characteristically, the patient will contrive a complex justification for his or her overreaction to what often appears to be a rather minor provocation. This pecularity, like the inclination to harbor grudges, appears to distinguish the temporal lobe epilepsy patient's aggressive/assaultive behavior from that observed in patients with frontal lobe lesions.

In reviewing the association of aggressive behavior and epilepsy, Taylor[36] has noted an increased prevalence of disturbed and disrupted home environments as contributing factors. Based on my own experience and numerous accounts by other authors, it seems clear that these critical environmental stimuli are more or less specific in each case. Thus they appear to trigger the angry outbursts in an almost reflex manner. That is, they appear to be conditioned or learned responses. It is well established that the limbic system plays a key role in learning and memory, and in mediating aggressive behavior.[37] Accordingly, it is suggested that epileptogenic foci, with their proclivity to establish abnormal, functional neuronal connections, appear to be uniquely situated, when they are located in or propagate to the temporal lobes, to elicit aberrant associations between these functions.

Inter-ictal Disturbances of Sexuality

There are a variety of problems related to the epilepsy patient's psychosexual adjustment and performance. Although, as indicated previously, these problems are less dramatic than ictal sexual difficulties, they occur more frequently.

Hyposexuality. A reduction in libido, *hyposexuality*, is the most frequently encountered inter-ictal sexual disturbance. Hyposexuality and other sexual disorders are probably much more common in epilepsy patients than is generally appreciated. There are at least two reasons for this. One is that despite certain attitudinal changes towards a more open discussion of problems related to sexuality, patients are often reticent about initiating such discussions with their physicians, many of whom are ignorant of or do not recognize the importance of such problems in their epilepsy patients. A second reason is that, because many cases of epilepsy begin before puberty, these patients may not recognize their own hyposexuality and therefore express no concern about it.

It is frequently stated that the reduced libido in epilepsy is nonspecific and simply reflects the more general psychosocial problems common to patients with chronic diseases of any sort. At variance with this suggestion, however, are several pieces of evidence. Gastaut and Collomb[38] noted that hyposexuality was seen only in temporal lobe epilepsy patients and was not observed in patients with idiopathic epilepsy. Moreover, hypersexuality, although less common, may occur in some epilepsy patients, a feature which is extremely rare in other chronic debilitating diseases.

It is also commonly believed that hyposexuality is related to taking anticonvulsant medications. The lack of a clear correlation between serum anticonvulsant levels and decreased sexuality argues against this suggestion. Similarly, when anticonvulsants bring about a reduction in seizure frequency there may be an equal increase in sexual drive. Moreover, hyposexuality may disappear following successful surgical treatment of epilepsy even when anticonvulsant medications continue to be taken postoperatively.[39]

Homosexuality. In a series of patients with medically intractable temporal lobe epilepsy, Blumer and Walker[40] noted a homosexual orientation in nearly 10 percent of their cases. The specificity of this relationship appeared to be confirmed by the appearance of a heterosexual adjustment following temporal lobectomy.

Fetishism and Transvestism. Fetishism and transvestism associated with temporal lobe epilepsy have been reported by many authors. In some cases[41, 42] the patients were said to have had no other manifestations of epilepsy. In some, their seizures appeared only many years after the onset of the transvestism and fetishism. Despite this, the EEG was abnormal in all cases. The patient reported by Mitchell et al.[43] is particularly noteworthy because his fetishistic act (viewing the point of an "unhooded" safety pin), which produced a feeling of sexual excitement, is linked to reflex epilepsy, a disorder that bridges the inter-ictal and ictal forms of epilepsy-related disturbances of sexuality. Following temporal lobectomy, the fetish and the seizures ceased, and this patient resumed satisfactory sexual relations with his wife. Thus the results of surgery appear to support the concept of a specific relationship between the epilepsy and the sexual disorder.

Epilepsy Type and Sexual Disturbances. In animals the central role played by the limbic system in mediating sexual behavior has been firmly established. It is probable that the hypersexuality demonstrated by Kluver and Bucy[44] in the temporal-lobectomized (destructive lesions) monkey has its counterpart in the hyposexuality seen in humans with temporal lobe epilepsy (irritative lesions). It is likely, too, that in humans influences arising in other parts of the brain, particularly the frontal cortex, play an important role in modulating and modifying limbically mediated sexual behavior. Based on these inter-ictal disorders and the ictal disturbances of sexuality, it appears that there is a fairly high degree of specificity regarding the type of epilepsy and the type of disordered sexuality. Thus epilepsy-related, complex disturbances of sexuality have, for the most part, a different neuroanatomical substrate from those simpler seizures primarily manifested by sensory phenomena localized to the erogenous zones. In the former, the epileptogenic focus is almost invariably located in some portion of the limbic system, particularly the temporal lobes. In the latter, the situation is more variable, but for the most part the epileptogenic focus in such cases is located in the vicinity of the paracentral lobule.[45]

Psychosis and Epilepsy

Of the various forms of psychopathology associated with epilepsy, perhaps the most serious is a schizophrenic-like psychosis. In an extensive report, Slater, Beard, and Glithero[46] have presented an excellent analysis of this disorder. In this, they detail the clinical findings in 69 patients in whom there was an association of epilepsy with a paranoid, schizopheniform psychosis. Of their 69 patients, 45 were cases of TLE. The authors point out that one distinguishing feature between this disorder and "true schizophrenia" appears to be the preservation of affect.

There is, of course, no reason why this schizophreniform psychosis of epilepsy should be exactly like the functional psychosis we call schizophrenia; but the important point is that on balance the psychoses are more alike than different. In an elaborate statistical study of this association, Guerrant et al.[47] set out to test the hypothesis that "people with *psychomotor epilepsy* are more disturbed psychiatrically than those with other chronic illnesses." They found that the frequency of psychosis among their psychomotor epileptics (all of whom had temporal lobe EEG foci) was five times that of their non-psychomotor group, that is, epileptics without demonstrable EEG foci. They attach little significance to this because 13 percent of their control group, made up of patients with "chronic medical illnesses," were also said to be psychotic—certainly a most unusual finding on a general medical service. In the end, however, the authors conclude their study by noting, "It cannot be said that the hypothesis was completely disproved." In point of fact, their epileptic and the non-epileptic (chronic-medical-illness) groups revealed many differences when specific psychopathological features were individually considered.

An interesting inverse relationship between the seizure frequency and the severity of this associated psychosis has been observed by other authors.[48,49] It is likely that it was this reciprocal relationship between the severity of the psychosis on the one hand and the seizure frequency on the other that lead to the mutual antagonism theory of Meduna,[50] which, through a curious translation, has come to be considered a theory of mutual exclusion. A parallel reciprocal relationship was noted by Landolt[51] in the EEG findings of these patients. Based on this he introduced the concept of "forced normalization." He used this term to denote the reduction of the EEG paroxysmal activity during a psychotic episode and the tendency for it to reappear at an equal rate with a decrease in the psychotic behavior.

As indicated above, the schizophrenic-like psychosis reported by Slater et al. occurred predominantly in their patients with temporal lobe epilepsy. Our own data[52] support this special association with TLE. Moreover, we noted that this paranoid schizophrenic-like psychosis and aggressive behavior both tend to occur more often when the epileptogenic focus involves the *left* temporal lobe. The specificity of this association with regard to laterality is in agreement with the earlier report of Flor-Henry.[53] Establishing the specificity of the relationship of certain forms of psychopathology to the laterality of the epileptogenic focus is complicated by the fact that scalp-EEG findings may be grossly misleading (see pages 92-93). Therefore, we recently re-examined[54] the specificity of this association, that is, left TLE with a schizophrenic-like psychosis, in a group of patients who had undergone depth electrode implantation as part of an evaluation for temporal lobectomy. We found 7 cases with unilateral epileptogenic foci, established with sufficient certainty to justify temporal lobectomy, who, in addition, had a history of a schizophreniform psychosis. Five of these 7 patients had left, and 2 patients right, temporal lobe foci, $p < 0.01$. Consistent with and supporting this concept that a left temporal lobe focus may be selectively associated with this schizophreniform psychosis are the observations of others[55,56] that there is a disproportionately large percentage of left-handers among such cases. In a like manner, certain of the specific personality traits occurring in some temporal lobe epilepsy patients appear to be related to the side of their epileptogenic focus.[57]

In summary, the studies cited indicate that when psychopathology supervenes in temporal lobe epilepsy it may take the specific form of a paranoid, schizophrenic-like psychosis. This association of a schizophreniform psychosis with TLE seems most likely to occur when the epileptogenic focus involves the left temporal lobe, and women appear to be at greater risk. The psychosis usually appears several years after the onset of the epilepsy and may begin following successful surgical treatment of the seizures.

HYSTERICAL SEIZURES AND TEMPORAL LOBE EPILEPSY

A frequently troublesome differential diagnostic consideration is the hysterical seizure (see Chapter 2) with its many manifestations. It might seem reasonable that malingering or feigned grand mal and focal epileptic seizures would be diagnosed by electroencephalography. From what has preceded, it should be clear that a normal EEG does not necessarily rule out the presence of a seizure disorder. In practice, it is uncommon to obtain an ictal EEG in such patients. When this is accomplished, the record is usually as obscured by artifact as an actual ictal (major-motor) tracing. Although hysterical attacks are held to depend upon unconscious mental mechanisms and feigned attacks are, by definition, consciously determined, in practice the two types are usually quite similar in appearance. Moreover, as difficult as the distinction between hysterical (or feigned) attacks on the one hand and true seizures on the other may be, even more perplexing is the patient who exhibits both types of attacks. This curious situation was recognized by Charcot, who described it as "hystérie à crises combinées." The causal factors underlying feigned attacks may be obvious, and to a lesser degree this may also be true for hysterical attacks. However, why some patients should exhibit such attacks in addition to genuine seizures is not obvious.

Diagnosis of the hysterical nature of an attack often depends upon demonstrating that the attack fails to make anatomical sense. That is to say, the clinical progression of the attack is not in accord with established neuronal connectivity. Experimental epilepsy in animals, however, reveals that abnormal, antidromic conduction occurs when the electrical fields (generated by multiple neurone discharges) excite axons as they pass through an epileptogenic focus. As a result, abnormal patterns of neuronal propagation occur that might account for many of the unusual seizure patterns seen in such patients. Similarly, such abnormal propagation might account for the failure of fibre sectioning operations (such as comissurotomy) in the treatment of epilepsy.

That notwithstanding, the important fact to keep in mind is that the patient presenting with what appears to be a bizarre (hysterical) seizure may in fact be suffering from true epilepsy. In my own experience, the combination of the two is most frequently encountered in patients with temporal lobe epilepsy.

THE EEG AND TEMPORAL LOBE EPILEPSY

It seems fair to say that in no other field has the original promise of electroencephalography for the diagnosis of brain dysfunction been realized more fully than in epilepsy. Despite this, it is variably estimated that upwards of 20 to 40 percent of patients with epilepsy, particularly temporal lobe epilepsy, have a "normal" routine electroencephalogram (EEG). As a result, electroencephalographers have been challenged to seek provocative techniques for eliciting diagnostic discharge patterns in the EEG of such patients. The large number of techniques that have been recommended, particularly for temporal lobe epilepsy, attest to the fact that this challenge has not been fully met. Sleep, either naturally occurring or pharmacologically induced, appears to be the most effective of these techniques. Short-acting barbiturates have been suggested as being particularly useful for activating the EEG of epilepsy patients. Our own studies[58] indicate that this has no superiority over natural sleep. However, sleep per se appears to be of definite, albeit limited, value and should be employed when the routine EEG is not diagnostic.

When epileptiform activity does occur, those electrical discharges which are deep in the temporal lobe frequently go undetected in the scalp-recorded EEG. Consequently, special, that is, nasopharyngeal and sphenoidal electrodes are sometimes used. In cases where surgical treatment of the epilepsy is contemplated, electrodes may be implanted deep within the brain parenchyma. Such explorations reveal that the conventionally recorded scalp-EEG frequently fails to disclose the epileptic focus or may be grossly misleading with respect to revealing the laterality of the focus.

Comparing depth and surface EEGs, Gloor, Oliver and Ives[59] found that at least 25 percent of the pre-implantion EEGs were false localizing. More disconcerting still are the findings in a recent study[60] comparing the localization predicted by depth recorded inter-ictal data and seizures provoked by electrical or chemical stimulation with the actual (spontaneous seizure) focus. They disclose that in at least one-third of the cases, the inter-ictal EEG data were misleading in indicating the laterality of the focus. Moreover, the degrees to which electrically and chemically induced seizures correlated with the laterality of the spontaneous seizure discharges were only 77 and 64 percent respectively.

It should be clear, therefore, that great caution must be exercised in drawing conclusions about the relationship of observed behavioral disturbances and the presumed laterality of the epileptogenic focus based on surface EEG data or even inter-ictal depth electrode data. These are disappointing but, of course, not unexpected findings. Obviously, although there can be no question that there is a fundamental relationship between physiological brain dysfunction on the one hand and disturbances of behavior on the other, it would be unreasonable to anticipate that this relationship would manifest itself in a one-to-one correlation of EEG data and behavior. This is particularly so when, as is usually the case, electrodes are implanted in only a limited number of sites. Because of this, the significant electrical events which might correlate with complex behavior may well be occurring at locations remote from the recording electrode(s). For example, in temporal lobe epilepsy with aggression it is conceivable that the electrical events that might relate to aggressive behavior may be occurring in the hypothalamus. Therefore, it is quite unlikely that the electrodes implanted in the temporal lobe itself would record the significant electrical correlates of such behavior. Moreover, since a single anatomical structure may contain several closely spaced zones of independent electrogenesis,[61] it might be necessary to implant multiple electrodes in a given target. It is possible, too, that such electro-behavioral discrepancies may derive, in part at least, from the important contribution made by the structural lesion underlying the electrical focus. This is supported by our observation[62] that pneumoencephalographically demonstrated abnormalities of the temporal lobes were better correlated with the behavioral disorders than were the EEG changes. Complementary studies involving Computerized Axial Tomography and Positron Emission Scanning will no doubt help to shed additional light on this relationship.

CONCLUSIONS

In this chapter, the complex and highly specific relationships between various forms of psychological dysfunction and different types of epilepsy have been explored. The data clearly indicate the necessity for obtaining a thorough and detailed psychological history on each epilepsy patient. It seems certain that, as a greater awareness of the association of psychopathology and epilepsy develops, so, too, will greater insights into the specificity of these relationships. Careful analysis of such relationships will undoubtedly help to insure a more thorough and complete evaluation of the epilepsy patient. Rather than stigmatizing the patient, an open and frank consideration of his or her psychological problems will have a healthy impact, leading to a more comprehensive treatment program.

REFERENCES

1. Temkin, O. *The Falling Sickness*, 2nd ed., Baltimore: John Hopkins Press, 1971, p. 467.
2. Lennox, W. G. *Personality and the Behavior Disorders*, J. McV. Hunt (ed.) Vol. 2, New York: Ronald, 1944, pp. 938-67.
3. Parsonage, M. Discussion of: Inter-ictal manifestations of complex partial seizures. In: J. K. Penry and D. D. Daly (eds.), *Advances in Neurology*, Vol 11, New York: Raven Press, 1975, pp. 111.
4. Epilepsy Foundation of America, Basic statistics on the epilepsies, Philadelphia: F. A. Davis, 1975, p. 61.
5. Masland, R. L. Commission for the control of epilepsy (guest editorial), *Neurology* 28:861-3, 1978.
6. Sontag, S. *Illness as Metaphor*. New York: Farrar, Straus and Giroux, 1978, p. 87.
7. Reynolds, E. H. Discussion of: Inter-ictal manifestations of complex partial seizures. In: J. K. Penry and D. D. Daly (eds.), *Advances in Neurology*, Vol 11, New York: Raven Press, 1975, p. 110.
8. Falret, J. De l'état mental des épileptiques. *Arch. Gen. de Med.* 16:661-79, 1860.
9. Morel, B. A. *Traites des mentales*. Paris: Librarie Victor Masson, 1860, p. 866.
10. Samt, P. Epileptische irreseinsformen. *Archiv für Psychiat. und Nervenkrank.* 6:110-216, 1876.
11. Gibbs, F. A. Ictal and non-ictal psychiatric disorders in temporal lobe epilepsy, *J. Nerv. Ment. Dis.* 113:522-8, 1948.
12. Ibid.
13. Jasper, H. H., Pertuisset, B., and Flanigin, H. EEG and cortical electrograms in patients with temporal lobe seizures. *Arch. Neurol. & Psychiat.* 65:272-90, 1951.
14. Gibbs, 1948, op. cit.
15. Stevens, J. R. Inter-ictal clinical manifestations of complex partial seizures. In: J. K. Penry and D. D. Daly (eds.), *Advances in Neurology*, Vol. 11, New York: Raven Press, 1975, pp. 88-112.
16. Penfield, W. and Jasper, H. *Epilepsy and the Functional Anatomy of the Human Brain*. Boston: Little, Brown and Co., 1954, pp. 409-10.
17. Stepien, J. S., Cordeau, J. P., and Rasmussen, T. The effect of temporal lobe and hippocampal lesions on auditory and visual recent memory in monkeys. *Brain* 83:470-89, 1960.
18. Scoville, W. B. and Milner, B. Loss of recent memory after bilateral hippocampal lesions, *J. Neurol. Neurosurg. Psychiat.* 15:99-107, 1957.
19. Talland, G. A. and Waugh, N. C. *The Pathology of Memory*. New York: Academic Press, 1969, p. 292.
20. Mullan, S. and Penfield, W. Illusions of comparative interpretation and emotion. *Arch. Neurol. & Psychiat.* (chic) 81:269-84, 1959.
21. Temkin, 1971, op. cit.
22. Hooshmand, H. and Brawley, B. W. Temporal lobe seizures and exhibitionism. *Neurology* 19:1119-24, 1969.
23. Freemon, F. R. and Nevis, A. H. Temporal lobe sexual seizures. *Neurology* 19:87-90, 1969.
24. Currier, R. D., Little, S. C., Suess, J. F., and Andy, O. J. Sexual seizures. *Arch. Neurol.* 25:260-4, 1971.
25. Erickson, T. Erotomania (nymphomania) as an expression of cortical epileptiform discharge. *Arch. Neurol. Psychiat.* 53:226-31, 1945.
26. Forel, A. *The Sexual Question: A Scientific, Psychological, Hygienic and Sociological Study*, 2nd ed., (Marshall, C.F., trans.) New York: Redman, 1911, p. 536.
27. Bancaud, J., Favel, P., and Bonis, A. Manifestations sexuelles paroxystiques et épilepsies temporale. Étude clinique, EEG et SEEG d'une épilepsie d'origine tumorais, *Rev. Neurol.* 123:217-30, 1970.

28. Hoenig, J. and Hamilton, C. M. Epilepsy and sexual orgasm. *Acta Psychiatr. Scand.* 35:448-56, 1960.
29. Meyer, L. Uber mania transitoria, *Virchow's Arch*, 8:192-210, 1855.
30. Monroe, R. R. *Episodic Behavioral Disorders.* Cambridge: Harvard University Press, 1970, p. 517.
31. Elliot, F. A. The neurology of explosive rage. The dyscontrol syndrome, *The Practitioner* 217:51-9, 1976.
32. Monroe, R. R., Balis, G., and Lion, J. R. Implication of findings. In: R. R. Monroe (ed.), *Brain Dysfunction in Aggressive Criminals*, Lexington, MA: Heath, 1978, pp. 165-173.
33. MacDonald, J. M. *Psychiatry and the Criminal.* Springfield, IL: C. C. Thomas, 1969, p. 352.
34. Knox, S. J. Epileptic automatisms and violence. *Med. Sci. Law* 8:96-104, 1968.
35. Gunn, J. and Fenton, G. Epilepsy, automatism and crime. *Lancet* 1:1173-6, 1971.
36. Taylor, D. C. Aggression and epilepsy. *J. Psychosom. Res.* 13:229-36, 1969.
37. MacLean, P. *A Triune Concept of the Brain and Behavior.* Toronto: University of Toronto Press, 1973, p. 165.
38. Gastaut, H. and Collomb, H. Étude de comportement sexuel chez les épileptiques psychomoteurs, *Ann. Med. Psychol.* 112 657-96, 1954.
39. Peters, U. H. Sexualstorungen bei psychomotorischer epilepsie, *J. Neurovisc. Relations. Suppl.* 10:491-7, 1971.
40. Blumer, D. and Walker, E. Sexual behavior in temporal lobe epilepsy—Effects of temporal lobectomy on sexual behavior. *Arch. Neurol.* 16:37-43, 1967.
41. Epstein, A. W. Relationship of fetishism and transvestism to brain and particularly temporal lobe dysfunction. *J. Nerv. Ment. Dis.* 133:247-58, 1961.
42. Hunter, R., Logue, V., and McMenemy, W. H. Temporal lobe epilepsy supervening on longstanding transvestism and festishism. *Epilepsia* 4:60-65, 1963.
43. Mitchell, W., Falconer, M. A., and Hill, D. Epilepsy with fetishism relieved by temporal lobectomy. *Lancet* 267:626-30, 1954.
44. Kluver, H. and Bucy, P. C. Psychic blindness and other symptoms following bilateral temporal lobectomy in rhesus monkeys. *Am. J. Physiol.*, 119:352-3, 1937.
45. Erickson, 1945, op. cit.
46. Slater, E., Beard, A. W., and Glithero, E. The schizophrenia like psychoses of epilepsy (i-v), *Brit. J. Psychiat.* 95:109-50, 1963.
47. Guerrant, J., Anderson, W. W., Fischer, A., Weinstein, M. R., Jaros, R. M., and Deskins, A. *Personality in Epilepsy.* Springfield, IL: C.C. Thomas, 1962, p. 112.
48. Yde, A., Lohose, E., and Faurbye, A. On the relation between schizophrenia, epilepsy and induced convulsions. *Acta Neurol. Psychiat. Scand.* 16:325-88, 1941.
49. Hachiya, H. Epileptic psychosis with schizophrenia-like manifestations: A clinical and genetic study. *Psychiat. Neurol. Jap.* 62:991-1011, 1960.
50. Von Meduna, L. General discussion of the cardiazol therapy. *Am. J. Psychiat. Suppl.* 94:40-50, 1938.
51. Landolt, J. Uber verstimmungen, dammer-austande und schizophrene zustandsbilder bei epilepsie. *Schweiz Arch. Neurol. Psychiat.* 76:313-21, 1955.
52. Sherwin, I. Clinical and EEG aspects of temporal lobe epilepsy with behavior disorder, the role of cerebral dominance. *McLean Hosp. J. Special Issue.* June: 40-50, 1977.
53. Flor-Henry, P. Schizophrenic like reactions and affective psychoses associated with temporal lobe epilepsy: Etiological factors. *Am. J. Psychiat.* 126:148-52, 1969.
54. Sherwin, I. Psychosis associated with epilepsy: Significance of the laterality of the eliptogenic lesion. *J. Neurol. Neurosurg. and Psychiatr.* 44:83-85, 1981.
55. Jensen, I. and Larsen, J. K. Mental aspects in drug resistant temporal lobe epilepsy. (abstract), *10th Epilepsy International Symposium*, Vancouver, Canada, 1978, pp. 196-7.
56. Kristensen, O. and Hein Sindrup, E. Psychomotor epilepsy and psychosis (I. Physical Aspects). *Acta Neurol. Scand.* 57:361-9, 1978.
57. Bear, D. M. and Fedio, P. Quantitative analysis of interictal behavior in temporal lobe

epilepsy. *Arch Neurol*. 34:454-67, 1977.
58. Sherwin, I. and Hooge, J. P. Comparative effectiveness of natural sleep and methohexital, provocative tests in electroencephalography. *Neurology* 23:973-6, 1973.
59. Gloor, P., Oliver, A., and Ives, J. Prolonged seizure monitoring with stereotaxically implanted depth electrodes in patients with bilateral interictal temporal epileptogenic foci: How bilateral is bitemporal epilepsy? (abstract) *10th Epilepsy International Symposium.* Vancouver, Canada, 1978, p. 22.
60. Wieser, H. G., Bancaud, J., Talairach, T., Bonis, A., and Szilka, G. Comparative value of spontaneous and chemically and electrically induced seizures in establishing the lateralization of temporal lobe seizures. *Epilepsia* 20:47-59, 1979.
61. Brazier, A. B. Spread of seizure discharges in epilepsy: Anatomical and electrophysiological correlates. *Exp. Neurol.* 36:263-72, 1972.
62. Sherwin, 1977, op. cit.

4

SPECIFIC PSYCHIATRIC COMPLICATIONS IN CERTAIN FORMS OF EPILEPSY AND THEIR TREATMENT

DIETRICH BLUMER, M.D.

Different forms of epilepsy tend to have very different effects on the mind of the afflicted—if, indeed, they have any effects at all.[1-6] Infantile epileptic encephalopathy (West Syndrome) and to a lesser degree the childhood epileptic encephalopathy (Lennox-Gastaut Syndrome) tend to be associated with intellectual deterioration. These are seizure disorders associated with marked cerebral damage. On the other hand, the common generalized seizure disorders such as petit mal or grand mal uncomplicated by any cerebral damage tend to have a benign course as far as the seizure disorder is concerned and are typically not associated with any significant and specific mental changes. Among the partial seizure disorders, cortical motor and sensory seizure disorders tend to be free of significant mental impairment, while the partial complex seizures originating from the limbic temporal lobe area are, by fairly general agreement, associated with a wealth of psychiatric changes, which vary from mild peculiarities of personality and behavior to severe and disabling mental changes, including psychosis.

If one looks for characteristic mental changes associated with epilepsy, it cannot be a surprise that temporal lobe epilepsy, with its chronic excessive and irregular neuronal discharges in the center of the limbic system, must be singled out. One must, however, keep in mind that seizure disorders which on the surface appear generalized in nature may carry signs of focal involvement (history of brain damage, neurological or neuroradiological findings, focal component to seizure or to EEG); they may have to be classified as generalized seizure disorder with either primary or secondary temporal lobe involvement and would carry a similar risk for psychiatric complications

97

as pure temporal lobe epilepsy. This applies particularly to the more intractable, not so benign "generalized" seizure disorders.

THE SIGNIFICANCE OF TEMPORAL LOBE INVOLVEMENT

Since the first half of the nineteenth century, the *ammonshorn sclerosis* has been recognized as an important pathological finding among institutionalized persons with epilepsy.[7] In the early 1950s, Henri Gastaut and his coworkers described specific behavioral changes among temporal lobe epileptics, which were absent among generalized seizure patients and could be viewed as traits of a partial inverse Klüver-Bucy Syndrome (Table 1).[2-4,6,9] These were, indeed, the same traits which were already well known to all psychiatrists dealing with institutionalized seizure populations. Considerable confusion reigned in the American literature, as long as the specific traits

Table 1

Syndrome of Temporal Hyperconnection

Hypometamorphosis	Viscosity
	\
	\Hypergraphia
	/Verbosity
	/
Hyperemotionality	Increased emotional depth
	Irritability-Anger-Rage
	Emotional lability—Mood Swings
	Goodnatured-Helpful Attitude
	Sense of Justice
	Religious (Philosophical)
	Interests
Hyposexuality	Decrease of sexual interest and arousal

This Table represents a partial elaboration of the behavioral syndrome described by Gastaut[8] and is referred to as *Syndrome of Temporal Hyperconnection*[17]. The syndrome of temporal hyperconnection in epilepsy represents a partial inverse Klüver-Bucy syndrome: the excessive tendency to attend immediately to each new stimulus perceived (hypermetamorphosis) stands in contrast to the excessive tendency to adhere to each thought, feeling and activity (hypometamorphosis or viscosity); tameness and lack of fear are in contrast to irritability and deepened emotionality, excessive sexual arousal to decreased erotic and genitopelvic arousal and response.

The sometimes very sticky adherence to each particular ongoing activity, feeling or thought and the deepened emotionality combine in the manifestation of heavy, prolonged (at times very ponderous) verbosity and hypergraphia.

were not clearly identified, and as long as it was not understood that many so-called generalized seizure patients also had a history of and/or the subtle changes characteristic of primary or secondary temporal lobe involvement.[10, 11] Rodin has recently shown[12] that a more severe mental impairment is characteristic of those temporal lobe epilepsy patients who also have generalized seizures. The role of concomitant generalized seizures present in perhaps one-half of temporal lobe epileptics (or of the infrequent frontal seizure activity) still needs further clarification. Such generalized seizures document the facilitation of spread from the focal discharge, and this factor may well play a role in the degree of expression of the mental changes.

Personality and behavioral changes, in various degree, tend to emerge some two years after onset of the temporal lobe seizure disorder and are a common finding. The more severe psychotic disorders are less common complications, occurring, when they do, on the average, some 14 years after the onset of epilepsy.

The mental effects of either focal or more diffuse brain damage associated with a seizure disorder (for example, frontal lobe damage) must be separately assessed. The specific effects of an active temporal lobe seizure disorder per se can be well appreciated if one considers that a very subtle lesion in the mesial limbic temporal lobe area can bring about a seizure disorder, and that many of the mental changes associated with temporal lobe epilepsy may be reversed upon ablation of the entire tip of a temporal lobe. The toxic or idiosyncratic effects of anticonvulsant medication on mental functions in a given individual have to be carefully considered, and can be usually distinguished by the experienced clinician from the specific mental changes related to the presence of chronic seizure activity. Of greater practical and theoretical significance than the direct effect of the anticonvulsant drugs on the mental state is their indirect effect via modification of the seizure disorder.

Changes Specific for Chronic Temporal Lobe Seizure Activity

At the risk of a certain amount of simplification, we will, then, discuss the mental changes specifically associated with temporal lobe epilepsy or epilepsy with temporal lobe involvement, and their treatment. They represent the most important psychiatric complications associated with the epilepsies.

The changes can be grouped as follows:

I. Primary Changes Specific for Chronic Temporal Lobe Seizure Activity.
    1. Behavior and Personality Changes
        a. Viscosity
        b. Deepened Emotionality

      c. Hyposexuality
   2. Mood Changes
   3. Psychoses
   4. Memory Disorders
II. Secondary Changes Frequently Associated With (But Not Specific For) Chronic Temporal Lobe Seizure Activity
   1. Hysterical Seizures (Hystero-Epilepsy)
   2. Depressive, Hypochondriacal and Hypomanic Traits
   3. Sensitivity and Paranoid Traits

These changes are discussed below.

I. Primary Changes

1. *Behavior and Personality Changes.* What the experienced observer terms merely a peculiar comportment can be clearly related to the three major character changes associated with chronic excessive neuronal discharges in the mesial temporal lobes and adjoining areas:[13] viscosity ("hypometamorphosis" or adhesiveness); deepened emotionality;[14] and hyposexuality.

a. *Viscosity.* Although the old concept of an "epileptic personality" has been largely discarded, the viscosity or "stickiness" that was considered its trait remains a sign of character disorder. Patients with this symptom tend to proceed laboriously and emphatically in their conversation or writing, bent on clarifying every detail.[15,16] Their talk may seem incoherent, branching out from the direct line of thought—yet they will stubbornly get back to and complete the original thought if permitted to do so. They tend to be verbose and have a marked difficulty in terminating a conversation. As a result, they may be shunned.

These patients tend to be viscous in all their behavior, and some clinicians contend that they can recognize the temporal lobe epileptic by his or her intense and prolonged handshake. A patient of ours complained bitterly that his boss would avoid him even though he talked with each of the other employees when he would visit the shop. It became evident that our patient had taken the friendly gesture of his boss very seriously, involving him in tediously long elaborations whenever he was given an opening. As a matter of expedience, the boss soon chose to pass him by.

We do not know of any drug that improves viscosity. Even successful surgical removal of an epileptogenic focus, with full control of seizures and normalization of EEG, does not seem to lead to an appreciable lessening of this trait. However, in some patients, viscosity can be overcome, at least to a degree, by gentle insistence and by reconditioning them to a more expedient form of verbal exchange. A too-passive interviewer will spend much time and obtain limited information. Of therapeutic importance is the fact that an intelligent patient can be confronted with his or her problem in communicating once a good rapport is present, and may learn to be more to the point and therefore more socially acceptable. It is possible that patients with chiefly left temporal epileptogenic focus tend to be more self-critical and therefore more willing to accept criticism from others, while patients with right temporal focus tend to deny their difficulties[17] and will be less open towards confrontation with problem traits such as viscosity.

b. *Deepened emotionality.* The detail-bound and long-winded manner of speech of many temporal lobe epileptics tends to be heavily laden with emotional emphasis and may assume a very ponderous nature. The increased depth of emotionality, in fact, appears to contribute to the viscosity, in that every single detail tends to become overly important.

We consider as the core of this deepened emotionality the hyperethical attitude commonly found among temporal lobe epileptics. Issues of right or wrong are central to them at all times; nothing can be taken too lightly, and sobriety prevails. The patients tend to fluctuate between a highly good-natured, helpful, often hyperreligious attitude, and briefer episodes of heightened anger, moodiness, or explosiveness, in the form of intense verbalized anger and threatened physical violence. These negative phases are soon followed by return of the good-natured attitude with much remorse—or, in other patients, with denial of their own negative behavior.[18] Some patients maintain a highly good-natured attitude throughout and others display explosive behavior only very rarely; however, many patients tend to fluctuate markedly between the opposite poles of being angry and hateful and being good-natured and helpful. One cannot understand temporal lobe epilepsy patients unless one understands this basic conflict. The writings of Dostoevski, the most famous temporal lobe epilepsy sufferer, consistently reflect this polarity between good and evil, crime and punishment, the saint and the murderer. The contrast strikes some observers as hypocritical, as Freud has noted.[19] In our opinion, both poles of the personality are genuine, and the good-natured side tends to be prevalent. However, it is for their angry outbursts that these patients lose friends, become at times intolerable to their families, and may be admitted to a psychiatric unit.[20,21]

One of our patients illustrates this syndrome. An unemployed young male with temporal lobe epilepsy as a result of a childhood lead encephalopathy, he was very slow, circumstantial, and ponderous in his conversation. He lived with his parents and spent much of his time in the courts, watching how justice was rendered. He also was very religious, yet prone to displays of excessive temper. One of his worst outbursts occurred when he was playing the same religious hymn over and over again on his stereo, until his father finally asked him to stop it. The patient was so enraged by this request that he began to destroy the furniture and had to be escorted by police to an emergency room.

Dangerous violence occurs very rarely in persons with epilepsy and tends to be confined to the confused post-ictal states of certain patients, which they do not remember afterwards.[22] The common inter-ictal irritability of the usually good-natured epileptic is relatively harmless, but nevertheless can reach very disturbing proportions. In children in particular, a reduction of anticonvulsants and allowance of more seizures may at times be necessary to reduce their irritability. Tegretol, in our experience, has an emotionally calming effect and can reduce an undesirable irritability to tolerable levels. The additional use of antipsychotics may be necessary, perhaps only at times of heightened irritability. On an investigational basis, we have treated chronic temporal lobe epileptics with excessive irritability with Depo-Provera and noted a significant calming effect.[23]

On the other hand the good-naturedness and religiosity associated with temporal lobe epilepsy may be considered positive changes, although sometimes an exaggerated helpfulness may be awkward or even intrusive to others.

c. *Hyposexuality.* Perhaps a majority of patients with temporal lobe epilepsy develop a global hyposexuality characterized by lack of interest in sexual matters and rare genital arousal.[24] This hyposexuality is a primary phenomenon if onset of temporal lobe epilepsy occurred before or at the time of sexual maturation, and is secondary if it develops upon later onset of temporal lobe epilepsy. The globally hyposexual patient is not bothered by his or her lack of interest in sexual matters and infrequency of sexual arousal. With late onset of seizures, the ensuing hyposexuality may be a troubling matter. On rare occasions, temporal lobe epilepsy patients may develop not only hyposexuality but a sexual interest in unusual matters (paraphilias).

It has been reported that temporal lobe epilepsy patients have been cured of fetishism and transvestism as well as of epilepsy by unilateral temporal lobectomy.[25,26] Some patients experience renewed sexual interest. A male patient with right temporal lobe epilepsy since age 13 had never experienced any kind of sexual arousal until the age of 30. At that time he underwent a successful right temporal lobectomy. Sexual arousal began to occur six months after surgery. He subsequently got married and would have intercourse with his wife every night even at the age of 40.[27]

A few temporal lobe epilepsy patients show some sexual arousal shortly after their seizures (post-ictal sexual arousal).[28] Rarely, if this occurs in the more immediate post-ictal phase, it may lead to inappropriate sexual behavior, with no subsequent recollection. An occasional patient may show sexual arousal during his or her seizures (ictal sexual arousal), experiencing or displaying a marked sexual component with the other symptoms. It is clear, however, that in the majority of patients with temporal lobe epilepsy the presence of chronic excessive neuronal activity in the mesial temporal lobes is associated with suppression of sexual arousal.

It is incorrect to blame anticonvulsant medication for the hyposexuality. Rather, with sufficient control of the seizure activity by medication, a revival of sexual interest and genital arousal may occur. The same phenomenon can be observed, sometimes dramatically, weeks or even months after successful unilateral temporal lobectomy. The hyposexuality is not a social problem, and thus often escapes medical attention. However, it leads to further social isolation of many persons with epilepsy (particularly those of the male sex), who do not feel compelled to seek sexual companionship and often tend to remain single.

2. *Mood Changes.* Frequently temporal lobe epilepsy patients will complain of rapid mood changes consisting of rapid cycling, within the same day, between hours of deep depression and briefer moments of elation. This lability of mood appears to occur particularly among adolescent and young patients and is a phenomenon not documented in the literature.

On the other hand, the longer-lasting *episodic* mood changes characteristic for epilepsy patients have been well described since Kraepelin. They consist of dysphoric episodes lasting for hours or days.[29,30] They are characterized by a fairly distinct onset, as the customary good-natured and considerate comportment changes to a brooding, tense, and irritable demeanor lasting for hours or days. Outbursts of anger may become increasingly likely and the patient's relatives may bend over backwards to avoid such a reaction. In a few patients these episodes may have rather a hypomanic character; in many one notes a marked sensitivity which may reach paranoid proportions. The episodes may terminate with a clinical seizure to be followed by exemplary (and remorseful) behavior. They may become more prevalent when the incidence of seizures has abated.

The episodic mood changes merely may represent accentuations of the characteristic "two-faced" personality of patients with temporal lobe epilepsy. On the other hand, they are akin to and may be precursors of the more severe disturbances that are labeled *intermittent psychoses.*

3. *Psychoses.* A psychosis following not a single attack but a flurry of seizures used to be common in the past (Table 2). This *post-ictal psychosis* is characterized by a brief lucid interval between a series of seizures and onset of a delirious state. It may last for days or as long as a couple of weeks. Since more effective anticonvulsants have been available, the post-ictal psychosis has become rare. Treatment is that of a delirious state and may often require antipsychotic medication.[1]

In modern times, the much more common psychosis associated with epilepsy is that *schizophrenia-like psychosis,*[31] which is characterized by a clear state of consciousness, occurs inter-ictally, sometimes terminating with a seizure, and often, perhaps in a third of the cases, occurs at times when seizures have become controlled (*alternating psychosis*).[5,13,32,33] These psychoses may occur after many years (average of 14 years) of epilepsy with temporal lobe involvement and may show any of the symptoms of schizophrenia, except that the basic personality is not schizoid. The emotionality is not flat but rather intense, and the rapport which the patient is able to establish remains surprisingly intact. The psychoses develop, then, in individuals with the familiar, more or less marked personality and mood changes of the temporal lobe epileptic. The course may be intermittent or

Table 2

Psychoses in Epilepsy

Inter-ictal	alternating with presence of epileptic manifestations; non-alternating	schizophrenia-like (basic personality is epileptoid, not schizoid)
Post-ictal	onset several hours to 48 hours after flurry of seizures	delirious
Ictal	petit mal status	stuporous
	temporal lobe status	delirious

To Landolt's original classification we have added the temporal lobe status, a diagnosis which is rarely made. Post-ictal psychoses (postepileptic twilight states) were common as long as effective anticonvulsants were not available. The inter-ictal psychoses have become better known with the era of modern anticonvulsants and may be either spontaneous or iatrogenic (occurring when seizure control is achieved by medication).

chronic, but without the deterioration that can be observed in schizophrenics.

Treatment may consist of Tegretol and/or antipsychotic drugs. If the psychosis is alternating in type, occurring for instance upon the introduction of a more effective anticonvulsant, then this particular offending drug should be discontinued, or anticonvulsant drugs may have to be reduced. On occasion, after careful assessment of all factors involved, the anticonvulsant medication may be stopped to allow for recurrence of seizures and remission of the psychosis. Rarely, a few ECTs may be employed in order to treat the psychosis with artificially induced seizures.

A case history illustrates the nature of the schizophrenia-like psychosis. A 45-year-old single woman had suffered from generalized seizures since the age of eight. In her early twenties she began to experience episodes of sudden sounds, which reached such a crescendo manner that she would be unable to speak or perceive. Each episode had an aftermath lasting perhaps a few minutes.

The woman had always lived with her parents, had never been interested in the opposite sex, but had been able to maintain a simple job steadily. While very religious, softspoken and good-natured in general, she could be, at times, very irritable and verbally abusive towards her mother, with whom she had remained after her father's death and her siblings' marriages.

Soon after her mother's death, the woman became more depressive. She lost her job. Her siblings would not visit her very often. She began to hear voices outside her windows, commenting on her actions or berating her harshly. These hallucinations occurred very frequently. In addition, she also began to hear buzzing and ringing sounds (which appeared to be related to her Tegretol). She finally decided she couldn't take her illness, the voices, and the noises anymore, and attempted to hang herself in the basement; she was saved when the rope broke.

She was then hospitalized. With moderate doses of antipsychotic medication, she gradually improved. She remained extremely shy and unable to get a job, but improved when her sisters and brothers began to make more efforts to visit her.

The stuporous state of a *petit-mal status* (spike-wave stupor), sometimes lasting for hours, has been listed among the psychoses associated with epilepsy,[34] but is a rather distinct entity. More difficult to recognize is a *temporal lobe status*.[5] This entity is rare but has to be kept in mind if one encounters an epilepsy patient with sudden onset of bizarre, incoherent behavior, unresponsiveness, confusion, and interspersed, repetitive and stereotyped manifestations of a temporal lobe seizure event (for example, oral automatisms). A mild form of temporal lobe status in which consciousness is not lost is the phenomenon of a *continuous aura*,[35] probably less rare than the more severe temporal lobe seizure status. EEG recordings clarify the diagnosis, and treatment with increased doses of anticonvulsants is indicated.

4. *Memory Disorders.* The temporal lobe seizure or any seizure with temporal lobe involvement is usually associated with a distinct memory impairment.[36] Even some patients who merely report an aura—that is, do not experience a lapse in the continuity of their awareness—may suffer a lapse in memory. Older people, in whom the capacity to remember has weakened, are particularly vulnerable. The more severe the seizure discharge, the more marked will be the memory lapse, and it is plausible that with bi-temporal involvement this lapse will be more protracted. If a series of seizures occur at short intervals, there may be a very prolonged amnesia, covering entire days.

Typically, there is an initial retrograde amnesia following a temporal lobe seizure. This amnesia shrinks fairly promptly as the patient regains his or her orientation and begins to recall what happened before the attack—except for a variably brief permanent retrograde memory gap. The post-ictal amnesia does not clear up, since no memorizing took place in that phase. Some patients get over their post-ictal confusion, can resume a simple conversation or routine activity, yet will not recall this phase. A few, post-ictally, may carry out perfectly appropriate and even complex actions for 15 minutes or longer, yet, to everybody's surprise, without any recall.[37] The so-called psychomotor automatisms are almost entirely phenomena of the post-ictal phase.

II. Secondary Changes

Some mental changes are frequently present in patients with temporal lobe epilepsy but are not specific for the condition. These traits are referred to as *secondary* mental changes. Their presence has further clouded the issue of specificity of the psychiatric complications of the epilepsies. We can simply state that their frequent presence demonstrates a high risk for development of manifold psychiatric changes, apart from the primary changes just discussed, in epilepsy patients with temporal lobe involvement.

Hysterical Seizures (Hystero-Epilepsy). Hysterical seizures, or pseudoseizures, are common among persons with epilepsy. But if we have patients with clearly hysterical seizures, we should always suspect that they may also have at least a mild genuine seizure disorder. We have frequently found a history of rape or sexual abuse among females with severe hysterical seizures, and this may be a significant finding.

Treatment is that of benign neglect of the hysterical attacks and of focusing on the emotional and interpersonal difficulties.[13,38] This may have to take place on a psychiatric inpatient unit. If anticonvulsants are increased because of incorrect diagnosis, this may result in a toxic state with increased primitive-hysterical manifestations.[39] EEGs often cannot be reassessed until one month from withdrawal from anticonvulsants, since barbiturate withdrawal is associated with abnormal findings. Patients with concomitant genuine seizure disorder need to be continued on modest doses of anticonvulsants.

Fugues in a dissociative state may also occur in persons with epilepsy. They have to be differentiated from the rarer cases that are motiveless and based on prolonged seizure activity.

2. *Depressive, Hypochondriacal and Hypomanic Traits.* Depression becomes an increasingly frequent finding in older epilepsy patients with temporal lobe involvement, as anger and aggression become less outward-directed.[40] In some, this occurs with successful treatment of the seizures with anticonvulsants. Tegretol or antidepressants may be helpful in controlling the depression. Occasionally there may be a need to allow some seizures for relief of a serious depression; this would seem preferable to the more artificial intervention with ECT in such patients. The suicide risk is higher among older temporal lobe epilepsy patients and, paradoxically, is particularly high at a time when the seizures have become controlled.[41] This contrasts with the occasional patient who makes a serious suicide attempt early, upon realization that he or she suffers from seizures which are disrupting his or her life. Hypochondriacal preoccupations are not uncommon and reflect a mild depressive state.

A few temporal lobe epilepsy patients show a persistent hypomanic comportment, which usually requires no special treatment.

3. *Sensitivity and Paranoid Traits.* A sensitive disposition and moderately paranoid attitudes may be chronically present. They are not pervasive. It is surprising how the same patient who relates very well to certain favorite persons may be very sensitive and react in a paranoid manner toward others; this occurs often when the person has not been treated with patience and consideration. The increasing isolation of many patients with epilepsy tends to favor this attitude.

Conclusion

Psychoses associated with epilepsy are not common events. The incidence reported varies between 2 percent and 30 percent, depending on the nature of the population studied. Personality and behavior changes are the rule rather than the exception with temporal lobe involvement of some severity and duration. The changes may remain rather subtle and to the casual observer may consist of merely a positive personality variant, for example, that of a good-natured, considerate, and conscientious human being. But many temporal lobe epilepsy patients become gradually "different" or "peculiar," and their social adjustment suffers.

The conclusion can be made that not only the seizures but also the described mental changes specifically found in temporal lobe epilepsy patients often lead to social isolation. These patients are basically friendly, emotional, and highly ethical people. Yet their emotional intensity and their overemphatic and overconscientious manner of conversing may not be so easily tolerated by others. Also, because of their irritable moods they may be shunned by others—or they may themselves choose to avoid others. They may feel more intensely about religious matters than the other parishioners or even the pastor, and they may choose to keep their thoughts about God and the universe to themselves. The reduced sexual interest favors another type of isolation, causing patients to avoid intimate contact with the opposite sex.

In psychosis, the isolation becomes most manifest, even though the patient tends to remain remarkably able to reach out for contact with a friendly human being.

Individuals with the traits characteristic for epilepsy with temporal lobe involvement need understanding, at least on the part of family and the helping professions, of their particular difficulties. They may require more friendly patience than is commonly afforded. Efforts at reeducation for the viscosity may have to be undertaken. Obviously, the maintenance of family ties and the securing of job opportunities are of utmost importance for the well-being of these patients.

REFERENCES

1. Blumer, D. Temporal lobe epilepsy and its psychiatric significance. In: F. Benson, D. Blumer (eds), *Psychiatric Aspects of Neurologic Disease*, New York: Grune and Stratton, 1975.
2. Gastaut, H., Roger, J., and Lesèvre, N. Differenciation psychologique des épileptiques en fonction des formes electrocliniques de leur maladie. *Revue De Psychologie Appliquée*, 3:237-249, 1953.
3. Gastaut, H. and Collomb, H. Etude de comportement sexual chez les épileptiques psychomoteurs. *Annales Médico-Psychologiques*, 112:657-696, 1954.
4. Gastaut, H., Morin, G., and Lesèvre, N. Etude de comportement des épileptiques psychomoteurs dans l'intervalle de leurs crises; les troubles de l'activité globale et de la sociabilité. *Annales Médico-Psychologiques*, 113:1-27, 1955.

5. Janz, D. *Die Epilepsien*, Stuttgart: G. Thieme, 1969.
6. Niedermeyer, E. *The Generalized Epilepsies*. Springfield, IL: C.C. Thomas, 1972.
7. Gastaut, H. Etat actuel des connaissances sur l'anatomie pathologiques des épilepsies. *Acta Neurologica Et Psychiatrica Belgica*, 56:5-20, 1956.
8. Gastaut, H. Interprétation des symptômes de l'épilepsie "psychomotrice" en fonction des données de la physiologie rhinencephalique. *Presse Medicale*, 62:1535-1537, 1954.
9. Klüver, H. and Bucy, P. C. Preliminary analysis of functions of the temporal lobe in monkeys. *Archives of Neurology and Psychiatry*, 42:979-1000, 1939.
10. Small, J. G., Small, I. F., and Hayden, M. P. Further psychiatric investigations of patients with temporal and nontemporal lobe epilepsy. *American Journal of Psychiatry*, 123:303-310, 1966.
11. Stevens, J. R. Psychiatric implications of psychomotor epilepsy. *Archives of General Psychiatry*, 14:461-471, 1966.
12. Rodin, E. A., Katz, M., Lennox, D. Difference between patients with temporal lobe seizures and those with other forms of epileptic attacks. *Epilepsia*, 17:313-320, 1976.
13. Blumer, D. Treatment of patients with seizure disorders referred because of psychiatric complications. *McLean Hospital Journal* (Special Issue), 53-73, 1977. See also Gastaut, op. cit.
14. Geschwind, N. The clinical setting of aggression in temporal lobe epilepsy. In W. S. Fields, and W. H. Sweet (eds), *The Neurobiology of Violence*, St. Louis: Warren H. Green, 1975.
15. Blumer, D., Benson, F. (eds) Personality changes with frontal and temporal lobe lesions. In: *Psychiatric Aspects of Neurologic Disease*. New York: Grune and Stratton, 1975.
16. Waxman, S. G. and Geschwind, N. Hypergraphia in temporal lobe epilepsy. *Neurology*, 24:629-636, 1974.
17. Bear, D. and Fedio, P. Quantitative analysis of interictal behavior in temporal lobe epilepsy. *Archives of Neurology*, 34:454-467, 1977.
18. Szondi, L. *Schicksalanalytische Therapie*, Bern, 1963.
19. Freud, S. Dostoevsky and parricide (1928). Strachey, E. (ed) Standard Edition Vol XXI, London, Hogarth, 1965.
20. Liddel, D. W. Observations on epileptic automatism in a mental hospital population. *Journal of Mental Science*, 99:732-748, 1953.
21. Roger, A., Dongier, M. Corrélations électroclinique chez 50 épileptiques internés. *Revue Neurologique*, 83:593-596, 1950.
22. Blumer, D. Epilepsy and violence. In: D. J. Madden and J. R. Lion (eds.), *Rage, Hate, Assault and Other Forms of Violence*, New York, Spectrum Publications, 1976, 207-221.
23. Blumer, D. and Migeon, C. Hormone and hormonal agents in the treatment of aggression. *J. Nervous Mental Dis.*, 160:127-137, 1975.
24. Blumer, D. and Walker, A. E. The neural basis of sexual behavior. In: F. Benson and D. Blumer (eds), *Psychiatric Aspects of Neurologic Disease*. New York: Grune and Stratton, 1975. See also Gastaut and Collomb, op. cit.
25. Mitchell, W., Falconer, M. A., Hill, D. Epilepsy with fetishism relieved by temporal lobectomy. *Lancet* 2:626-630, 1954.
26. Hunter, R., Logue, V., and McMenemy, W. H. Temporal lobe epilepsy supervening on long standing transvestism and fetishism. *Epilepsia* 4:60-65, 1963.
28. Blumer, D. Hypersexual episodes in temporal lobe epilepsy. *American Journal of Psychiatry*, 126:1099-1106, 1970.
27. Blumer, D. and Walker, A. E. Sexual behavior in temporal lobe epilepsy. *Arch. Neurol.* 16:37-43, 1967.
29. Slater, E. and Roth, M. *Clinical Psychiatry* (ed. 3). London: Baillière, Tindall, and Cassell, 1969.
30. Blumer, D. Psychiatric aspects of temporal lobe epilepsy: a review. In: J. A. Wada (ed.), *Epilepsy: Neurotransmitter, Behavior, and Pregnancy*, Joint Publication of Canadian League Against Epilepsy, Western Institute on Epilepsy, 1979.
31. Slater, E., Beard, A. W., and Glithero, E. The schizophrenia-like psychoses of epilepsy. *Br. J. Psychiatry* 109:95-150, 1963.

32. Bruens, J. H. Psychoses in epilepsy. In: O. Magnus and A. M. Lorentz De Haas (eds.), *The Epilepsies. Handbook of Clinical Neurology*, Vol 15. Amsterdam: North-Holland, 1974, 593-610.

33. Helmchen, H. Reversible psychic disorders in epileptic patients, 175–186. In: W. Birkmayer (ed.), *Epileptic Seizures—Behavior—Pain*. Bern-Stuttgart-Vienna: Huber, 1976.

34. Landolt, H. Serial electroencephalographic investigations during psychotic episodes in epileptic patients and during schizophrenic attacks. *Folia Psychiat. Neurol. Neurochir. Neerlandica Suppl.*, 4:9-133, 1938.

35. Scott, J. S. and Masland, R. L. Occurrence of "continuous symptoms" in epileptic patients. *Neurology* 3:297-301, 1953.

36. Blumer, D. and Walker, A. E. Memory in temporal lobe epileptics. In: G. A. Talland and C. Qaugh (eds.), *The Pathology of Memory*, New York: Academic Press, 1969.

37. Jackson, J. H. On a particular variety of epilepsy ("intellectual aura"), one case with symptoms of organic brain disease. In: J. Taylor (ed.), *Selected Writings of John Hughlings Jackson*, vol. 1. London: Staples Press, 1958, 399-405.

38. Rodin, E. A. Psychosocial management of patients with complex partial seizures. *Advances in Neurology*, 11:383-414, 1975. See also Blumer, 1977, op. cit.

39. Niedermeyer, E., Blumer, D., Holscher, E., and Walker, B. A. Classical hysterical seizures facilitated by anticonvulsant toxicity. *Psychiat. Clin.* 3:71-84, 1970.

40. Blumer, 1977, op. cit.

41. Janz, op. cit.

5

PSYCHOLOGICAL ASSESSMENT IN EPILEPSY

CARL B. DODRILL, PH.D.

Psychological evaluation of individuals with epilepsy has been done for many years, and one does not have to look far to determine why this is the case. For centuries it has been believed that some behavioral pattern generally characterized persons with epilepsy. An early statement of this was made by Aretaeus: "They become languid, spiritless, stupid, inhuman, unsociable, not disposed to hold intercourse, not sociable at any period in life; sleepless, subject to many horrid dreams, without appetite, and with bad digestion, pale, of leaden colour, slow to learn from the torpidity of understanding and of the senses."[1]

In recent years people have spoken of the "epileptic personality" (see Chapters 3 and 4) which is said to demonstrate many of these characteristics. As discussed in the earlier chapters of this book, such a view of individuals with seizure disorders is highly oversimplified, and it could hardly be expected that a group of disorders as complex as this would demonstrate universal psychological characteristics of any type. Evaluative procedures must therefore be equal to the complexities involved.

There are, in fact, a number of important topics involving psychological assessment that are of interest to the mental health practitioner. First, the very nature of the disease, with its intermittent and frequently unpredictable occurrence, places a series of stresses on the individual—stresses which, in many cases, have devastating emotional and social consequences. Secondly,

The preparation of this chapter and a portion of the research reported herein was supported by NIH Contracts NO1-NS-0-2281 and NO1-NS-6-2341, and by NIH Research Grant No. NS-02053, awarded by the National Institute of Neurological and Communicative Disorders and Stroke, PHS/DHEW. In addition, major development of the Washington Psychosocial Seizure Inventory was supported by a grant from the Epilepsy Foundation of America.

the nature of the disorder is such that the brain is necessarily involved. Since the brain is the seat of psychological abilities, and in most cases there are electroencephalographic abnormalities identifiable between attacks, it is reasonable to expect some disruption in cognitive processes. The products of these two groups of factors are so great that they very frequently exceed the effects of the seizures themselves, when adjustment to life is considered. Because of this, they constitute the two basic areas to be discussed here.

Epilepsy presents a different set of stresses to the individual than that seen with other disorders. While evaluative techniques developed with other groups can often be used, the unique problems encountered by the person with seizures are only very poorly assessed unless there is specific attention given to the problems associated with this disorder. Thus, the assessment approaches discussed in this chapter have been specifically developed for work with adults having seizure disorders.

ASSESSMENT OF PSYCHOSOCIAL FUNCTIONING

Clinicians working with individuals with epilepsy have observed numerous psychosocial difficulties. As one of America's foremost epileptologists has said, "There is practically no epileptic patient who is not confronted with some kind of psychosocial problem."[2] One does not have to look far to determine why this is the case. Social stigma, discrimination, and the tendency to associate epilepsy with demon possession are only a few of the factors which make life extremely difficult for the person having seizures. The intermittent appearance of the disorder tends to keep the people around the patient, as well as the patient him or herself, on edge. The casual observer soon knows what to expect of the individual with cerebral palsy, for example, but the person with epilepsy may change in behavior rather dramatically from one minute to the next—and for no apparent reason. Strange actions make everyone ill at ease, and it is easier not to associate with the seizure patient than to risk being caught in an embarrassing circumstance.

Despite the fact that the vast majority of individuals with epilepsy are under stresses of one sort or another, it is also commonly observed that such individuals vary substantially in the degree to which they are able to make a satisfactory adjustment to these stresses and to the demands of everyday life. In fact, it has often appeared that social factors are just as important in determining a person's ability to adjust to the demands of life as are seizures themselves, if not more so.

Development of the Washington Psychosocial Seizure Inventory (WPSI)

Because of the stresses that the person with epilepsy faces, along with widely divergent degrees of psychosocial adjustment, several of my colleagues at the Epilepsy Center and I developed an inventory to quantify aspects of psychosocial adjustment important to the person with seizures. In the development of such an inventory, we realized that systematic assessment would have to be provided in areas of importance for the adjustment of individuals with seizure disorders. After a considerable amount of work in the area, including pilot studies, we were able to identify seven important psychosocial areas, and these, together with an overall index, ultimately became scales of the Washington Psychosocial Seizure Inventory (WPSI):

1. *Family Background.* The foundation for later adjustment is laid in the home, and a patient's own response to seizures may well reflect the responses of family members. Thus, the inventory includes questions about relationships with family members, happiness and security in the home, and the extent to which it was believed that parents really cared for the individual in question. Questions in this area also pertain to relationships with peers during childhood and felt acceptance by school teachers. In short, the goal is to cover important interpersonal relationships during the childhood years as they might have a bearing on later adjustment.

2. *Emotional Adjustment.* Although there was no intention to develop a test containing detailed analyses of emotional problems, it was recognized that an overall indicator of emotional functioning was desirable. The vast majority of the problems covered pertain to neurotic or neurotic-like symptomatology, including depression, feelings of hopelessness and helplessness, generalized fatigue, worry, guilt, irritability, tension and anxiety, physical symptoms, and a general dissatisfaction with life. All of these problems have been frequently reported with individuals with epilepsy.

3. *Interpersonal Adjustment.* This area pertains to the extent of which subjects have healthy and meaningful contacts with others which can form a basis for good general adjustment. Questions pertain to the ease with which the individual establishes and maintains relationships, contentment with social contacts, the degree to which meaningful social relationships exist, anxiety in social situations, interpersonal trust, and general enjoyment of association with people. We were acutely aware that the extent to which an individual was adjusting appropriately to life hinged rather heavily upon ability to relate to other people.

4. *Vocational Adjustment.* The high unemployment rate among persons with epilepsy and the psychosocial consequences of such unemployment required attention. We therefore constructed a series of questions that dealt with vocational adjustment, particularly as it relates to seizures. Subjects are asked whether or not they would be in another line of work if they

did not have epilepsy, whether they have ever lost a job because of their seizures, whether they have problems in transportation, and in general if they are experiencing problems in the vocational area.

5. *Financial Status.* The questions in this area inquire from several perspectives whether or not the individual has enough money to meet basic needs and whether or not there is a feeling of financial security.

6. *Acceptance of Seizures.* A person's basic failure to come to grips with the reality of the seizure disorder has often been found clinically. Questions were therefore constructed pertaining to resentfulness of the seizures, embarrassment, dread of seizures, fear of rejection by others due to seizures, and general feelings of being able to cope with the attacks.

7. *Medicine and Medical Management.* In addition to the above areas, we were aware of the importance of the relationship between the physician and the patient, as well as whether or not the patient believed that the doctor was concerned, competent, likable, and making the best effort possible to control the seizures. Compliance in taking medications was also considered under this area.

8. *Overall Psychosocial Functioning.* An overall index of psychosocial adjustment was desired and this ultimately included considerations pertaining to the preceding seven areas but with a particular emphasis upon Emotional Adjustment.

In order to develop scales for each of the above areas, 127 adults with epilepsy were evaluated by the social service and psychology staff and by other people whose sole work was with individuals having seizure problems. By a series of ratings, it was possible to evaluate each patient for each area on an objective basis. By the point-biserial correlation technique, these professional ratings were then correlated with each of the 132 items that had been constructed. It was a priori determined that any item would be included in one and only one of the above scales, based upon purely statistical determinations; the item was to be included in the scale with which it correlated greatest, providing that the correlation was statistically significant at the .01 level or better. The development of these scales was crossvalidated. In addition, inter-rater reliability and test-retest stability studies were carried out, as were studies of validity. All of these studies are reported in the original paper.[3]

In addition to developing the clinical scales, we were very much aware that checks would be required on the extent to which the inventory was accurately and honestly completed. Three validity scales were therefore devised and are routinely scored for each inventory completed. The first merely consists of the number of items left blank or otherwise invalidated, and it was arbitrarily decided that if more than 13 of the items (10 percent) were not scorable, the profile would be considered invalid. Second, a Lie Scale was composed from a series of 10 items that ask about behaviors that are socially desirable but that are very rarely found. This is similar to the Lie Scale of the Minnesota Multiphasic Personality Inventory (MMPI). Of the 10 items in this scale, answering four or more in the Lie direction raises questions about the validity of the inventory. Finally, a Rare Item Scale was developed that was intended to parallel the F Scale of the MMPI which is discussed on pages 122-25. It ultimately consisted of 17 items, each of which was endorsed less than 15 percent of the time by subjects. Because all such rarely endorsed items are included in this scale regardless of content, the scale is highly diverse. By clinical work and by statistical estimation of the probability of endorsement of a series of these items, it was determined that when five or more are answered in the scored direction, questions about the validity of the Inventory should be raised.

The results of the scored WPSI can be plotted on a profile sheet. A sample of the profile sheet is presented in Figure 1. In developing the profile, linear regression techniques were used by which profile elevations were determined as a function of the professional ratings of difficulties in each area. Higher profile elevations identify greater problems. This system provides for a visual display of scores and the extent of difficulties appears to be roughly comparable from one area to the next when profile elevations are similar. To assist in interpretation, four areas of profile elevations are identified:

1. *No Significant Problems.* Scores here are routinely not accompanied by professional judgments of any difficulties.
2. *Possible Problems.* Scores here are occasionally associated with persons for whom professionals believe that some difficulties may exist, but where such problems are found they are routinely of limited significance.
3. *Definite Problems.* Scores here are associated with the identification of distinct and important problem areas in life as evaluated by the professional staff.
4. *Severe Problems.* Problems here are routinely identified by the professionals as being far-reaching and as having a striking impact on a person's ability to adjust to life.

With the above guidelines for interpretation in mind, one can now generally interpret the profile pattern plotted in Figure 1. This line corresponds to the mean scores of 199 adult epilepsy patients evaluated at our facility. In concert with our clinical judgment, the inventory identifies definite problems in several areas for the typical patient but finds emotional concerns to be at the forefront. With some degree of regularity, subjects consistently report uncertainties about themselves, aspects of depression, tension, anxiety, worry, and diffuse physical complaints. In addition, the typical patient demonstrates definite difficulties in dealing with others and may show de-

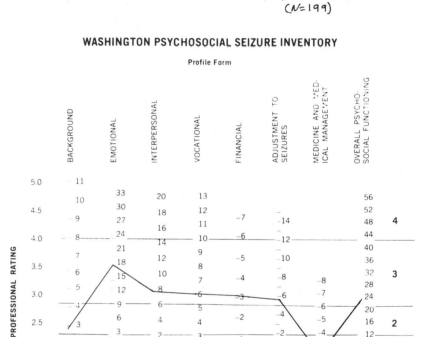

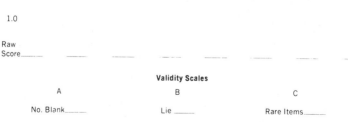

Figure 1. WPSI average profile for 199 adults with epilepsy

creased social skills. Problems in vocational adjustment are typically revealed which usually include the perception that the seizure disorder is relevant to such difficulties. As expected, financial concerns tend to exist as well. In addition, in spite of the fact that the majority of these individuals have had seizures for many years, problems in acceptance of the seizures themselves are in evidence for the average patient. With all these findings, it is not surprising that with the typical patient there are definite problems in overall adjustment.

Clinical Uses of the WPSI

A short series of WPSI profiles illustrating various types of adjustment in epilepsy will now be presented. Figure 2 gives the profile of J.S. This 35-year-old man had a WAIS Full Scale IQ of 142 and was working on this doctorate when he decided to become a fisherman in Alaska. He had temporal lobe or complex partial seizures as often as three times per day, but he made an excellent adjustment to the attacks and demonstrated no psychosocial problems. In fact, we would not have evaluated him at all were it not for his inclusion in the original study which required an unbiased sample of patients appearing on certain clinic days. As one can see from Figure 2, there are no elevations on this profile whatever. In addition, it should be observed that the Validity Scales were all within normal limits. Thus, this is an individual of whom we can be quite sure that there are no significant psychosocial problems, and the profile reflects what we saw clinically.

Figure 3 presents a case of very striking contrasts. This 23-year-old man has a history of chronic unemployment and severe dependency upon his mother, with whom he continues to live. He has a lifelong history of generalized tonic-clonic (grand mal) seizures, which began at age six months and continue to appear intermittently. Psychiatrically, this man demonstrates symptoms indicative of psychosis, including delusions of persecution, visual and auditory hallucinations, ideas of reference and inference, and feelings of unreality. This profound disturbance is reflected in the figure, where elements of his disorder are more prominently seen on the Emotional Adjustment and Interpersonal Adjustment scales. Further, the subject demonstrates striking failure to adjust to and to accept his seizure disorder. In addition, one should observe that his Overall Psychosocial Functioning Scale is in area 4, which indicates a most debilitating psychosocial condition. Even apart from his history, a WPSI profile of this type can only indicate profound psychological and psychosocial disturbance. Clearly, before any efforts can be made to place this man in a job situation or otherwise advance him, his emotional status must be dealt with and some alleviation of this condition must be realized. In this particular instance, his pathological relationship with his mother appears to require alteration before progress can be made in the emotional and interpersonal areas. Attempts were therefore made to change the relationship, but without success.

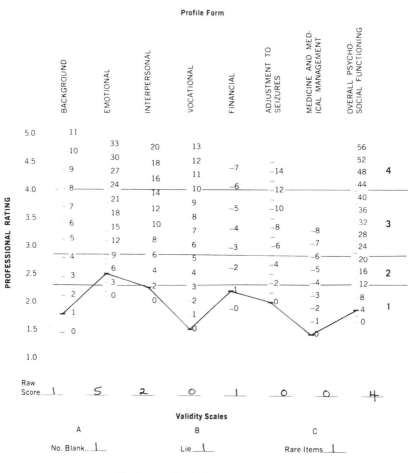

Figure 2. WPSI profile for an individual with no signs of psychosocial difficulties

An example of an individual with epilepsy but with predominantly neurotic symptomatology is presented in Figure 4. R.M. was a 34-year-old Caucasian man with nearly a college degree who had had recurrent seizures since age four. At the time he was seen in our Epilepsy Center, he was described by our social service staff as angry, frustrated, anxious, timid, mildly depressed,

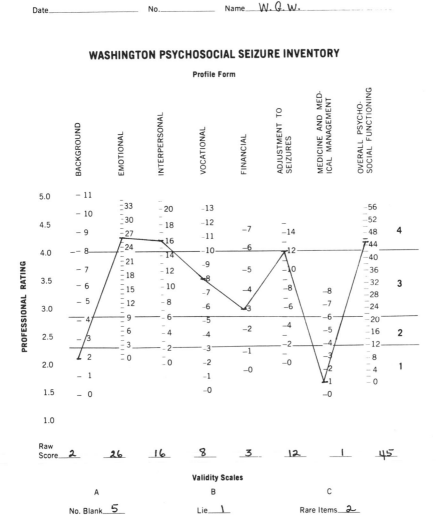

Figure 3. WPSI profile for an individual with psychosis and epilepsy

constricted, emotionally oversensitive, and having a flat affect. The MMPI was suggestive of multiple neurotic complaints, including depression, nervousness, anxiety, weakness, fatigue, social withdrawal, and a pervasive lack of self-esteem. There was, furthermore, the suggestion that psychological conflicts might be represented as physical complaints. When this type of

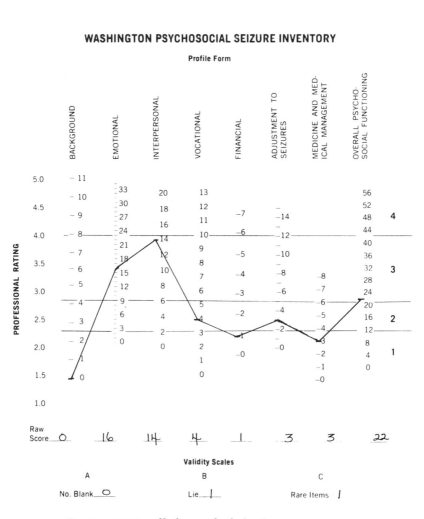

Figure 4. WPSI profile for an individual with neurosis and epilepsy

picture is uncomplicated by other psychological problems, elevations on the Emotional Adjustment and Interpersonal Adjustment scales are often seen as predominant, which is true in this instance. Furthermore, the overall level of maladjustment tends to fall in the third area instead of the fourth, indicating less severe difficulty. It was believed, however, that the problems this man demonstrated had a rather definite impact on his ability to adjust to everyday life, and it was therefore recommended that he be involved in the Social Skills Program of the Epilepsy Center in an effort to enhance his social and emotional functioning.

We now turn to an example of an individual with epilepsy who demonstrated a character disorder or psychopathic reaction. C.L. was a 27-year-old Caucasian female with a history of behavioral difficulties, including suspension from school, heavy alcohol use, use of many street drugs, and sexual permissiveness. She described herself as a "hell-raiser" throughout her life, though in recent years she had evidenced a little more stability. The MMPI was suggestive of a psychopathic or sociopathic reaction, although there were other factors in the profile, including somatic concerns, anxiety, and unusual trends in her thinking. She had had seizures since age 17. They consisted of myoclonic and major motor attacks. Her WPSI profile is seen in Figure 5 and it demonstrates a general pattern often seen in individuals with character disorders. There is evidence for defective relationships in the home in which she grew up, followed by later interpersonal concerns and evidence of rebelliousness. Note, for example, the relatively high score on the Medicine and Medical Management Scale, which clearly suggests difficulties in accepting direction from authority figures. Persons with scores of this type have often been noted to take their medications on schedules devised by themselves rather than by their physicians. Not only do they have trouble accepting the judgment of others, but they may have difficulty in accepting their epilepsy. When the felt need for employment as assessed by the Vocational Adjustment Scale is compared with that for money (Financial Status Scale), such individuals routinely demonstrate a greater need for the products of employment than for the work itself. Decreased motivation to work is thereby indicated, which is consistent with the inability to postpone gratification often seen with these people. The overall extent of maladjustment often falls in the third area.

The above cases illustrate various profile patterns. One should observe, however, that the typical patient does not have a stereotypic diagnostic pattern; in the usual instance, there are varying degrees of difficulties. In our clinical work with people having seizures, we have found that this Inventory helps us to more quickly identify areas of concern, which can then be explored in more detail in clinical interview and further testing. Treatment recommendations routinely follow.

ASSESSMENT OF PERSONALITY AND OF PSYCHIATRIC PROBLEMS

Emotional adjustment among persons with epilepsy is a topic that has
been of interest for many years. This is especially true when seizure disorders
are considered which involve the temporal lobes, for it is very commonly

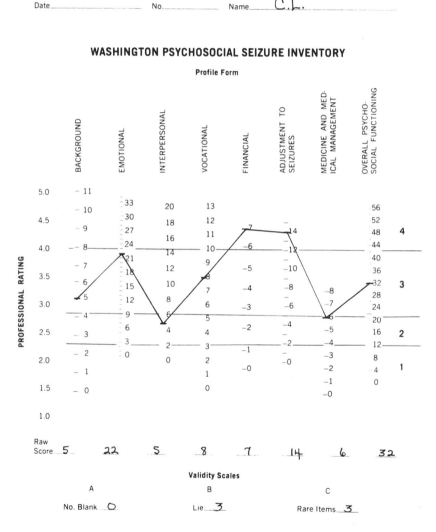

Figure 5. WPSI profile for an individual with a character disorder and epilepsy

believed that they are to be associated with emotional and behavioral alterations.[4,5,6,7] Objective support for such a position is not firm,[8] but interest in the area continues. While behavioral ratings and projective tests are often used to evaluate emotional status among persons with epilepsy, the advantages of objective procedures have not been missed. Because the Minnesota Multiphasic Personality Inventory (MMPI) is the most widely used inventory in this area, it will be discussed exclusively. One should be aware, however, that any of a large number of personality assessment procedures can and have been used with persons having epilepsy. Such procedures include those which are both objective and projective by nature, and many have no doubt been used successfully. The difficulty in covering them in more than a general descriptive way is that consistent and reliable patterns of performance have not appeared which are characteristic of epilepsy, and the research literature here tends to be fragmentary. They do constitute alternatives to either the WPSI or the MMPI, however.

The MMPI was originally devised to aid in making psychiatric diagnoses. The value of the procedure in psychiatric evaluation and treatment includes the extensiveness of the item pool, the richness of the clinical lore surrounding the various scales of the inventory, and the broadness of the research that has been done with it. There are, of course, liabilities associated with this inventory. They include its length, the large number of double negatives in the items, the objectionable nature of some of the content, and so on. The area to be discussed here, though, is the application of the MMPI to individuals having seizure disorders.

Undoubtedly, the biggest problem in applying the MMPI to persons with epilepsy is the large series of items whose content could be—or probably is—reflective of seizures themselves rather than of emotional disturbances. In temporal lobe, psychomotor, or partial complex epilepsy, seizures may manifest themselves in multiple ways so that many items on a scale such as "schizophrenia" may be endorsed. It would not be unusual for an individual with such attacks to endorse such items as "I have had periods in which I carried on activities without knowing later what I had been doing," "I am afraid of losing my mind," "I have strange and peculiar thoughts," "I have had more trouble concentrating than others seem to have," and "I have had attacks in which I could not control my movements or speech, but in which I knew what was going on around me." Certainly these phenomena would be viewed as unusual, if not frankly bizarre, in a psychiatric context, but their endorsement by a person having seizures would not necessarily indicate any psychological disturbance. Even when the seizures are minor attacks such as focal sensory or focal motor spells (elementary partial seizures), there are once again a number of items on the Schizophrenia Scale to which the individual might respond in the deviant direction: "I have never been paralyzed or had any unusual weakness of any of my muscles" (False), "I have little or no trouble with my muscles twitching or jumping" (False), "Once a week or oftener I suddenly feel hot all over, without apparent cause" (True), and "I have numbness in one or more regions of my skin" (False). The difficulty is that for persons without seizures these responses are peculiar and demand attention, whereas individuals with epilepsy may merely be reporting the substance of the attacks.

To illustrate how the above responses can affect profile patterns, the average profile of 50 adults with seizures given the MMPI is plotted in Figure 6. In my experience, this profile is characteristic of individuals having seizures who are experiencing a certain amount of stress as they face the problems of everyday life. The interpretation of the individual profiles with persons having seizures therefore becomes complex; this is especially true because of the likelihood that only a portion of the elevation on the Schizophrenia Scale can be attributed to the attacks themselves. In many instances, it is clearly apparent that persons with epilepsy do have some schizoid mentation which can in no way be considered to be a reflection of the attack itself. In the usual clinical interpretation, one generally deemphasizes to some degree elevations on such a scale while at the same time examining a detailed list of critical items to determine if there are endorsements which would appear *not* to be the result of the particular types of

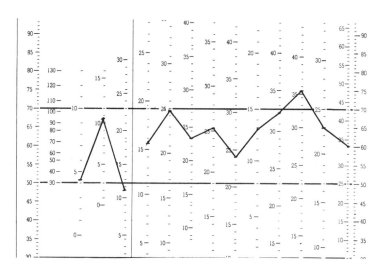

Figure 6. Mean MMPI profile for 50 adults with seizure disorders

seizures that the patient is experiencing. To a lesser degree also, some of the other scale elevations must take into account the particular seizure pattern demonstrated by the patient.

Using the above procedures, we have found that the MMPI is, and continues to be, a useful tool with epilepsy patients. It contains far more detailed evaluations of emotional status than is provided by the WPSI, and with the K Scale it provides a degree of sophistication with respect to the interpretation of profiles that is not yet possible with the WPSI. We thus continue to use the MMPI although we feel that the limitations identified above must be taken into account when it is applied to persons with epilepsy.

ASSESSMENT OF ABILITIES AND NEUROPSYCHOLOGICAL IMPAIRMENT

The evaluation of intelligence among persons with epilepsy has been of interest for many years; indeed, Turner presented an extensive review of the area in 1907.[9] Furthermore, whenever efforts have been made to evaluate the abilities of people with seizures, attention has most frequently been turned to intelligence, and formal assessment has often been made. Tarter[10] has presented a brief review of a series of studies in this area, almost all of which show persons with epilepsy to have slightly to substantially decreased intellectual abilities. The reasons for this are not hard to find. For one thing, epilepsy is a symptom of brain dysfunction. Even between attacks, there is evidence that the brain is not functioning well in the majority of people with seizures. These people tend to demonstrate abnormal electroencephalograms, including epileptiform discharges which are consistent with a diagnosis of seizure disorder. It is inconceivable that these abnormal wave forms would have no impact upon mental abilities, and therefore decreased intelligence should be expected. Additional factors such as social stigma and social isolation are frequently found which may have a variety of deleterious effects. Decreased performance under such conditions is likely.

Even though intelligence has been known to be related to neurological impairment, the discipline of clinical neuropsychology has now brought to light a number of factors of interest to professionals dealing with epilepsy. One of these factors is that intelligence tests are not sufficient measures of neurological impairment. Such tests were designed to determine how well a person could do in school; they were not deliberately constructed with items designed to be sensitive to problems in brain functions. Consequently, it is possible for an individual to do very well on a test of intelligence and still manifest impairment in brain functions or brain damage having a definite impact upon ability to adapt to the problems of everyday life. Brain functions are extremely complicated and diverse, so that a complete battery of tests is required to evaluate a range of functions if one is to have any hope of reflecting the behavioral and adaptive correlates of neurological disorders. Furthermore, in order to assure that the tests administered are sensitive to problems in brain functions, each test must have demonstrated validity and must differentiate individuals with and without neurological concerns. Factors such as these led Halstead[11] and Reitan[12] to develop a series of neurological tests whose goal is to identify problems in brain functions and ultimately their impact upon a person's ability to adapt to situations in everyday life. These tests are very well described in Reitan and Davison.[13]

The Neuropsychological Battery for Epilepsy

Beginning with the work of Halstead and Reitan, the present author developed a series of neuropsychological tests specifically for individuals having seizure disorders. As a stimulus to this work, it was recognized that persons with seizures could not automatically be assumed to be the same as those persons without such attacks. For one thing, the electrical changes generally associated with seizure disorders do have impacts on functioning.[14] For another, individuals with seizures take anticonvulsant medications on a chronic basis and these have been associated with certain deficits and inabilities.[15,16] In addition, there are areas of evaluation that appeared to be particularly important in epilepsy but that are not well evaluated by those tests in the Halstead-Reitan battery. These areas include memory and sustained attention to the task. Furthermore, only very incomplete and poorly documented norms have been established on the tests in the Halstead-Reitan battery and with individuals not necessarily having seizure disorders. Because of these factors and others, it was decided that it would be worthwhile to develop a group of tests specifically to evaluate brain-related deficits in individuals with seizure disorders and to standardize those tests on this particular patient group.

The battery of tests that was ultimately developed has been described in detail.[17] It will be reviewed here briefly, and a case will be described to illustrate the clinical application of the battery. From the start, it was recognized that two basic types of tests would be needed. First, a series of General Measures would be required that would evaluate areas of importance in clinical work but that would not be directed specifically to the problem of inadequate brain functions. With respect to adults, intelligence was one of the areas to be assessed, and it was decided that this would be evaluated by means of the Wechsler Adult Intelligence Scale (WAIS). Emotional adjustment was to be examined by the Minnesota Multiphasic Personality Inventory (MMPI). Preference in handedness was to be determined by Reitan's Lateral Dominance Examination.[18] Although other tests for each of these areas might have been chosen, these are recognized test procedures, and they were selected without additional evaluation.

Beyond the *General Measures* just identified, it was decided that a series of specific or *Discriminative Measures* would be required, each of which would point to problems in brain functions with people having seizures. To this end, three studies were sequentially run, including a pilot study, a principal investigation, and a cross-validational study. A total of approximately 100 neuropsychological measures were screened initially, and these were ultimately reduced to 16 test measures. No test measure was considered for inclusion unless it discriminated between control and epileptic persons at the .01 level or better. No test could overlap with any other test more than any one of Halstead's tests overlapped with any other of Halstead's tests (.66). Finally, each test measure had to demonstrate its ability to discriminate between normal and epileptic persons in a new cross-validational study. The 16 test measures finally selected became the Discriminative Measures of the Neuropsychological Battery for Epilepsy.

A brief description of these follows:

The Stroop Test. This consists of a modified form of the classical Stroop procedure. A single color plate is used in which color names are printed in incongruous colors ("red" is printed in green ink, "orange" is printed in blue ink, etc.). In the first part of this procedure, the person must simply read the words down the page as rapidly as possible and this alone became an effective discriminator between normal and epileptic persons. In the second part, the person must read the color of ink, ignoring the word. This is a very difficult test and requires a great deal of concentration. When Part 1 is subtracted from Part 2, a measure of "static" or interference is provided, and it is this latter variable which is the second Discriminative Measure.

Wechsler Memory Scale Form I. Two portions of the Wechsler Memory Scale were ultimately adopted as Discriminative Measures. The first consisted of the total number of memories from Logical Memory. The second consisted of the total score on the Visual Reproduction portion of the Scale. These measures provide assessment of verbal and non-verbal memory, and they help to evaluate an area of common complaint among persons with epilepsy.

Reitan-Kløve Perceptual Examination. This is the standard form of this test except that the portion involving the use of coins was omitted. Tests included assessment of tactual, auditory, and visual perception, as well as agraphagnosia, finger agnosia, and astereognosis. The total number of errors made on this test is the variable under consideration.

Name Writing Procedure. Originally, this came from the Lateral Dominance

Examination. As used in this battery, it consists of the calculation of the number of letters per second executed by the preferred hand, the non-preferred hand, and both hands taken together. The total score is the Discriminative Measure.

Category Test. This is the 208-item adult version of this problem-solving test, and it is given in the standard manner.[19]

Tactual Performance Test. This test is given in standard fashion as originally prescribed by Halstead, and the three indicators of functioning are preserved, including the Time Component, Memory Component, and Localization Component.

Seashore Tests of Musical Talents. The one test ultimately identified for use by Halstead and Reitan was included. This is the Rhythm Test. In addition, the Tonal Memory Test was included.

Finger Tapping Test. This also follows standard procedures used by Halstead and Reitan, except that the ultimate score identified as a Discriminative Measure consists of the individual performances of both hands combined.

Trail Making Test. Both Part A and Part B of this test are used, although it is only the number of seconds required to complete the latter part which is counted.

Aphasia Screening Test. A manual has been developed by which language errors can be identified, and the number of these errors is one of the 16 overall scores. In addition, criteria have been developed for evaluating constructional dyspraxia or distortion in visual-spatial relationships, and the final one of the 16 indicators springs from this.

For each of the above test measures, cut-off scores have been established that delineate normal and abnormal performance. An index is provided that identifies how many performances fall outside normal limits. Because of the large number of measures going into this single indicator, it has demonstrated great stability. For each person evaluated, the percentage of scores falling outside normal limits can easily be calculated and the extent of neurological impairment can be roughly estimated using the following standards: 0-30 percent = Normal Performance; 30-40 percent = Borderline Performance; 40-50 percent = Very Mild Impairment; 50-70 percent = Mild Impairment; 70-90 percent = Moderate Impairment; and 90-100 percent = Severe Impairment in brain functions. In addition to evaluating the test measures on the basis of general level of performance, it is, of course, possible to compare the relative performances of the right and left sides of the body and also to look for signs of specific neurological deficits that taken alone would be suggestive of impairment in brain functions.

Clinical Use of the Neuropsychological Battery for Epilepsy

C. H. was a 20-year-old Caucasian male who was referred for a neuropsychological evaluation by one of the counselors in the Vocational Unit of our Epilepsy Center. Approximately five years prior to evaluation he had been involved in a severe automobile accident that resulted in a depressed skull fracture on the right side of the head, with a two-month period of unconsciousness and a subsequent left hemiparesis. He has had major motor seizures for approximately the last three years. The referral was to determine his capabilities for the future, with particular reference to employment. The findings of the neuropsychological tests are summarized in Figure 7. A glance at the results of the WAIS indicates that this young man has average intellectual abilities overall, but that there is a substantial amount of variation from one area to the next with respect to his exact level of performance. As is true for perhaps 75 percent of people with seizure disorders, the Verbal IQ is greater than the Performance IQ, and this may in part be a reflection of the fact that the Performance Scale seems to be more sensitive to brain problems. At any rate, psychometrically he performs within the average range with respect to intelligence.

A review of the 16 specialized neuropsychological tests, however, clearly indicates that there are many signs of brain injury with this young man. In 12 of 16 cases (75 percent), his scores fall outside normal limits and in the range characteristic of the performance of individuals with impairing seizure disorders. Such a general level of performance is indicative of moderate impairment in brain functions. Furthermore, an examination of the scores of the particular tests administered reveals ample evidence for the brain injury, with both cerebral hemispheres probably being involved but the right cerebral hemisphere much more than the left. On the perceptual examination, for example, the subject made a total of 45 errors with respect to the left side of the body, but none at all with respect to the right side. His left hand was, in fact, so disabled that it was not possible for him to complete the Tactual Performance Test with that hand, and all three trials had to be done with the right hand. As one reviews the various tests, it is apparent that in every instance in which the left upper extremity is involved, there is substantial disability. This would have very strong implications for any vocational situation requiring the simultaneous use of both hands. In addition, it was observed that the subject had difficulties with other functions associated with the right cerebral hemisphere, including visual-spatial relationships and memory for nonverbal materials.

Language-related abilities fell inside normal limits. However, the subject's

NEUROPSYCHOLOGICAL REPORT--EPILEPSY CENTER

Name____C. H._____ Hospital No._____ Date_12/18/78____ No._826___

Age__20__ Education__12*__ Handedness__R__ Race_C_ Occupation__Student_____

NEUROPSYCHOLOGICAL BATTERY FOR EPILEPSY

Discriminative Measures

Note: Left hemiparesis

Stroop Test	Part I	144(2)*	Category Test		51
	Part II 250(5)	II - I 106			
			Tactual Performance Test		
Wechsler Memory Scale (Form I)			Preferred 15.0(5 in)	Total Time	(38.0)*
	Verbal (Stories)	13*	preferred 11.8(all in)	Memory	8
	Visual-Spatial (Drawings)	6*	Preferred 11.2(all in)	Localization	1*

Perceptual Examination

Seashore Rhythm Test   23*

Seashore Tonal Memory Test   17*

	R	L	
Misperceptions	0	(8)	
Suppressions	0	(8)	
Finger Agnosia	0	(10)	
Agraphagnosia	0	(15)	
Astereognosis	0	(4)	
Total Errors	0	(45)	(45)*
Astereo. Time	15	74	

Finger Tapping
    Preferred__35__ Nonpreferred_6___   41*

Trail Making Test
    Part A _42_   Part B   134*

Aphasia Screening Test
    Expressive__1__ Receptive_1___   2

Name Writing (Let/Sec)
    Pref._.90_ Nonpref._.12__   .21*

Constructional Dyspraxia   Mild*

*Performance falls outside normal limits. Total tests outside normal limits: 12/16 (75%)

General Measures

Wechsler Adult Intelligence Scale		Minnesota Multiphasic Personality Inventory		Lateral Dominance Examination	
VIQ _103_ Info _8_ Dig Sym_6_		? _50_ Pd _57_ Es _42_		R	L
PIQ _86_ Comp _15_ Pic Com_11_		L _50_ Mf _51_ Ep _23_		Hand _7_ _0_	
FSIQ _96_ Arith _10_ Bl Des _9_		F _55_ Pa _53_ A _7_		Eye _2_ _0_	
VSS _63_ Simil _13_ Pic Arr_6_		K _53_ Pt _44_ R _19_ Man		Foot _2_ _0_	
PSS _40_ Dig Sp_7_ Obj Ass_8_		Hs _62_ Sc _63_ Anx_8_		Dyna. _55.5_ _20.0_	
TSS _103_ Vocab _10_		D _48_ Ma _60_ Cr. _5_ In.			
		Hy _64_ Si _48_			

Figure 7. Neuropsychological profile for C.H., a 20-year-old Caucasian male with post traumatic epilepsy

ability to attend to the task and to perform in a sustained manner was less than would be expected, as revealed by the Seashore Rhythm Test and the Seashore Tonal Memory Test. Despite the obviously devastating effect that this brain injury has had upon his performance, it is of interest to note that his Category Test score is actually quite adequate and that his performance on the difficult part of the Stroop Test was also fairly good. Taken together, the neuropsychological tests point to definite signs of impairment in brain functions which, nevertheless, are quite lateralized and relate specifically to the right cerebral hemisphere and to the functions traditionally associated with that hemisphere.

Emotional status was evaluated by means of the MMPI. In many respects, this patient's performance on this inventory was within normal limits, although there was some suggestion of the use of repression and denial as a means of coping with psychological conflicts, and the possibility was raised that functional physical complaints may result from periods of prolonged emotional stress.

In the area of recommendations, focus was made almost entirely upon vocational placement. In making such recommendations, it was apparent that it would be desirable if a position could be found where the patient could use his verbal or language-related skills rather than relying primarily upon visual-spatial abilities. This is true not only because of his decreased visual-spatial abilities, but also because of the specific motor and sensory weakness that he demonstrates with respect to the left side of the body. Because he is a sociable individual with relatively intact language skills, a position that would involve both of these areas of strengths would appear to be most desirable. Because of some facial disfigurement following the accident and his obvious left hemiparesis, a position which does not require meeting the public on a face-to-face basis but in which he can use his verbal skills would appear ideal. The possibility of a telephone switchboard operator was especially recommended because it includes contact with other people, is unimanual by nature, and emphasizes language-related skills.

In general, it has been our experience that utilization of a full battery of neuropsychological tests is especially helpful in clients with definite neurological difficulties. With the individuals that we have seen, we have been able to identify in at least three of four instances neurological problems that are sufficiently severe to have detectable behavioral correlates. Even though we tend to see the more severely impaired individuals with epilepsy, it is our belief that the vast majority of persons with such a disorder do have some impairment in brain functions with impact for adjustment to everyday life. A neuropsychological evaluation appears to be an indispensable procedure in accurately evaluating the disabilities noted and in planning effectively for the future.

CONCLUSIONS

In this chapter, an effort has been made to present a review of assessment procedures particularly useful in dealing with the adult with epilepsy. Some of these procedures which seem to be of greatest value have been specifically designed for assessment in this context and are not merely procedures designed for other patient populations and applied to persons with seizure disorders. A complete evaluation of this type is a complex one, which typically requires a full day for the testing alone. However, because of the complexities demonstrated in brain functions and in social behavior, it appears that only through such an assessment can the full range of deficits be sought out and dealt with effectively.

REFERENCES

1. Temkin, O. The Falling Sickness. Baltimore: Johns Hopkins Press, 1945.
2. Rodin, E. A. Psychosocial management of patients with seizure disorders. McLean Hospital Journal. 1977, 74-85.
3. Dodrill, C. B., Batzel, L. W., Queisser, H. R., and Temkin, N. R. An objective method for the assessment of psychological and social difficulties among epileptics. Epilepsia, 21:123-135, 1980.
4. Flor-Henry, P. Psychosis and temporal lobe epilepsy: A controlled investigation. Epilepsia, 10:363-395, 1969.
5. Flor-Henry, P. Ictal and interictal psychiatric manifestations in epilepsy: Specific or nonspecific? A critical review of some of the evidence. Epilepsia, 13:767-772, 1972.
6. Flor-Henry, P. Psychosis, neurosis and epilepsy. British Journal of Psychiatry, 124:144-150, 1974.
7. Flor-Henry, P. Lateralized temporal-limbic dysfunction and psychopathology. Annals of the New York Academy of Sciences, 280:777-797, 1976.
8. Rodin, E. A., Kats, M., and Lennox, K. Differences between patients with temporal lobe seizures and those with other forms of epileptic attacks. Epilepsia, 17:313-320, 1976.
9. Turner, W. A. Epilepsy—A study of the idiopathic disease. London: Macmillan, 1907.
10. Tarter, R. E. Intellectual and adaptive functioning in epilepsy: A review of fifty years of research. Diseases of the Nervous System, 33:763-770, 1972.
11. Halstead, W. C. Brain and intelligence: A quantitative study of the frontal lobes. Chicago: University of Chicago Press, 1947.
12. Reitan, R. M. An investigation of the validity of Halstead's measures of biological intelligence. Archives of Neurology and Psychiatry, 53:28-35, 1955.
13. Reitan, R. M. and Davison, L. A. (eds.). Clinical neuropsychology: Current status and applications. Washington, D.C.: V. H. Winston, 1974.
14. Wilkus, R. J. and Dodrill, C. B. Neuropsychological correlates of the electroencephalogram in epileptics: I. Topographic distribution and average rate of epileptiform activity. Epilepsia, 17:89-100, 1976.
15. Dodrill, C. B. Diphenylhydantoin serum levels, toxicity, and neuropsychological performance in patients with epilepsy. Epilepsia, 16:593-600, 1975.
16. Dodrill, C. B. and Troupin, A. S. Psychotropic effects of carbamazepine in epilepsy: A double-blind comparison with phenytoin. Neurology, 27:1023-1028, 1977.
17. Dodrill, C. B. A neuropsychological battery for epilepsy. Epilepsia, 19:611-623, 1978.
18. Reitan and Davison, 1974, op. cit.
19. Ibid.

III.
THERAPEUTIC MEASURES

6

PSYCHODYNAMIC MANAGEMENT OF EPILEPSY

HARRY SANDS, PH.D.

Personality problems, social adjustment difficulties, conflicts—both conscious and unconscious—and the struggle to cope with the tasks of independent living all may give rise to tension and stress in persons with epilepsy. Anxiety and emotional stress arising out of these difficulties that exist without the individual's awareness of their precise nature are known to increase the frequency of seizures.[1,2,3] Such conflicts are "a sufficient sign for therapy in order to uncover the conflicts and to bring them into awareness since they also often play a role in the patient-doctor relationship and account for poor compliance [with the prescribed medical regime]."[4]

Such varying characteristics as age of seizure onset, types of seizures, degree of control, and seizure triggers are also related to psychological and social adjustment. The psychodynamic approach to the understanding of behavior takes into account all of these factors and their relative contributions in determining individual adjustment. In patients with epilepsy it provides a comprehensive picture of the way past and present factors in the individual's history are responsible for the patient's current problems and complaints. Thus, psychodynamic assessment draws on the neurological findings; on psychological factors, including cognition, learned conditioned responses, attitudes, developmental and intrapsychic factors; on social environmental factors, including interpersonal and economic; and on the spiritual factors, including ethnic and cultural. These identifiable components in varying combinations determine behavior. Wolberg refers to these factors as links in the behavior chain.[5]

This chapter will elaborate on these factors or links and will discuss the patient's history from the standpoint of developmental stages to identify each

135

factor and its relative contribution to personality development and adjustment in the patient with epilepsy. Also covered are the special considerations required to conduct dynamic short-term psychotherapy with seizure patients and the administration of educational and counseling techniques.

FACTORS INVOLVED IN ADJUSTMENT

In developing a treatment plan for the person with epilepsy, the mental health clinician must consider the patient's adjustment in these areas:

1. Patient's acceptance of and adjustment to seizures and the medical regime necessary to control them.
2. Patient's accommodation to the behavior resulting from the vicissitudes of the underlying neuronal activity.
3. Patient's manner of dealing with the emotional consequences of seizures and with the role of emotion and tension in triggering seizures.
4. Intrapsychic conflicts and the dynamic meaning of epilepsy for the patient.
5. Patient's reality testing and ability to cope with the demands of daily and independent living and with social and community reactions to epilepsy which at times can be barriers to employment, school, and other aspects of daily life.

To achieve the maximum effect of the therapeutic intervention, the mental health clinician must be able to assess the relative contribution of each of these factors to the psychological and social problems of the patient with epilepsy and the consequences for personal adjustment. The clinician must decide which factors require change and which cannot be changed but need to be compensated for in order to allow the patient's fullest use of his or her abilities and capacities for a productive and independent life in the community. As the Commission for the Control of Epilepsy and Its Consequences has stated:

> Our ability to provide appropriate counseling for people with epilepsy can be materially enhanced by the achievement of a precise understanding of the burden which epilepsy imposes on them, and through the establishment of means whereby destructive changes in behavior can be overcome.[6]

DETERMINANTS OF ADAPTATION IN PERSONS WITH EPILEPSY

A comprehensive treatment plan for the seizure patient starts with a psychodynamic understanding of the development of the patient and of the way he or she adjusts to epilepsy and its consequences. The plan focuses on the behavioral links which interfere with coping and adjustment mechanisms and which can be changed by therapy or, if they cannot be changed, at least be made to have less effect on coping.

Some problems which can be assessed psychodynamically are specifically associated with such characteristics as the age of seizure onset, the nature and frequency of seizures, the ictal (seizure) state, and the effects of anticonvulsant medications.

Age at Onset

The onset of seizures and the diagnosis of epilepsy have a profound impact on the person with epilepsy and his or her family. Arangio asserts:

> Whatever the age of onset, most patients and their families are in a heightened anxiety due to the occurrence of the first seizure. They are confused, baffled, fearful and perhaps panicked; their lives have been uprooted.[7]

Thus, the occurrence of the first seizure at any developmental stage is traumatic, and can interfere with subsequent normal personality development and result in adaptive breakdown and personality distortions.

As an example, the age-specific developmental tasks to be accomplished for normal personality growth at age six, when a child is about to enter school, are intellectual growth and understanding, further social contacts and organized team play, belonging to a group, club, or gang; the age-specific task to be achieved at this age is group identification.[8] The trauma caused by the onset of seizures at this time in development can give rise to symptoms such as adaptive breakdown, psychoneurotic reactions, anxiety states, phobic states, phobic reactions, primary behavior disorders, and juvenile schizophrenia; the resulting personality distortions are an inability to accept a proper role, disturbed relations with others, and problems in competitiveness and cooperation.[8]

It is therefore understandable that clinicians have thus hypothesized a positive relationship between the age of onset of seizures and specific adjustment difficulties. Tonic-clonic seizures beginning in early childhood have been linked to cognitive deficits.[8a] Temporal lobe seizures that start in adolescence have been reported to be positively related to psychopathology as measured by the Minnesota Multiphasic Personality Inventory (MMPI).[9] The duration of the seizure disorder is also related to lowered mental status and problems in adjustment.[10,11]

Seizure Characteristics

No one behavior or adjustment pattern has been agreed to as being characteristic of the different seizure types according to Sands and Price[12] and Feldman and Ricks[13] except for the often reported pre-ictal and post-ictal behavior associated with partial seizures in temporal lobe epilepsy (see Chapters 3 and 4).

However, many clinicians have observed that specific seizure characteristics can affect a patient's adaptation. Some of the more prominent seizure characteristics that may influence behavior are discussed below.

Aura. Patients who experience a sensory aura (see page 11) with sufficient time between it and the seizure use this warning to withdraw to a place of safety and seclusion to have their seizure, thus reducing the risk of being hurt or embarrassed. For many patients though, the aura is the actual onset of the ictal state and cannot serve as an aid to adjustment; rather it may signal fear of the oncoming seizure.

Pre-ictal Behavior. One of the more frequent pre-ictal behaviors is the shriek caused by the expulsion of air at the start of a grand mal seizure. The unexpected occurrence of the vocal outburst and its startling characteristic can be upsetting to others present—though not to the person having the attack, since he or she is anamnestic to it.

Some people cannot respond to others during the pre-ictal state; this behavior has caused some individuals to be seen as defiant and consequently manhandled by the police or, on rare occasions, arrested.

Ictal Behavior. Behavior during seizures has been discussed on pages 10-17. It should be noted that temporal lobe seizures can be disturbing to onlookers who do not realize that the person is having a seizure. Symptoms such as a failure to respond when talked to, grimacing movements of the mouth and face, smacking of lips and tongue, can be seen as bizarre. An even more severe social impact may be caused by the automatism of undressing or removing objects from tables and other furniture.

Post-ictal Behavior. Confusion, severe muscle aches, fatigue, drowsiness, sleep, and shame and embarrassment are the most frequent post-seizure behaviors that have bearing on the patient's adjustment.

Frequency of Seizures. Epileptologists have observed a clinical correlation between adjustment and the frequency of seizures. Thus, frequent grand mal, petit mal, or psychomotor seizures can have a more profound effect on adjustment to tasks of daily living than do less frequent seizures. A corollary is the degree of seizure control: the less control, the greater the adjustment problems. It is common to see patients depressed, frustrated, and hopeless as a result of not having gained control of seizures after much effort and compliance to an anticonvulsant drug regime.

Seizure Triggers. A number of stimuli are capable of precipitating seizures. They range from sensory stimuli to tension and emotional stimuli.[14]

Specific environmental antecedents to seizures are distinguished by their close time proximity to the seizures, and the reliability and predictability of this relationship between the stimulus-trigger and the ensuing seizure. The reflex type of epilepsy (see page 83) is an example of this kind of sensory seizure.

Visual stimuli are the most common sensory triggers. Other sensory seizure triggers include auditory, olfactory, and somatic stimuli. Complex stimuli patterns that induce seizures include music and voice.[15]

Stress has been implicated as a cause of seizure occurrences, although studies have not established a correlation between the objective signs of stress and clinical seizures.[16]

It has been shown, though, that acute anxiety, whether reactive to a reality situation or due to unconscious conflicts, can activate epileptiform discharges or clinical seizures. Thus, Lennox[17] described cases in which fear and anxiety have precipitated attacks.

Time and Place of Occurrence. The time at which a seizure takes place also affects adjustment. Nocturnal seizures occurring while the patient is asleep are likely to have less impact on adjustment than those occurring during the waking daytime hours. Similarly, seizures taking place immediately upon awakening have less effect on adjustment than do attacks during school or working hours.

The place where seizures occur may also be a factor in adjustment. Thus, a seizure that occurs while the patient is at work or in a public place has a greater impact than one that takes place at home.

Antiepileptic Drugs. Some side effects of anticonvulsant drugs have important consequences on personal adjustment. Masland notes (pages 34-40) that depression, drowsiness, dizziness, headaches, irritability, and hyperactivity are some of the side effects commonly associated with these drugs. Hirsutism in a girl or woman and gingival hyperplasia—both side effects of diphenyl-hydantoin (Dilantin)—and sexual impotence in some adults taking primidone (Mysoline) can result in severe psychosocial problems. Similarly, an ataxic gait or inarticulate or slurred speech as a result of drug toxicity are side effects that can be mistaken for drunkenness and substantially impair adjustment and coping.

Patient's Reaction to Seizures

A wide range of individual reactions to epilepsy have been observed in clinical practice. Some patients deny their seizures to the degree that they are non-compliant with their medical drug regime or carry on activities that, under conditions of uncontrolled seizures, can be dangerous—driving a car, scuba diving, mountain climbing, and so on. Other patients become withdrawn and fearful, some to the point of being shut-ins, out of shame or fear of having a seizure in public or of injuring themselves.

Seizures and Other Disabilities

The multiply disabled person with epilepsy has a more difficult task in coping and adjusting. The total disability is more than the mere sum of the two or more disabling conditions. Seizures and cognitive deficits due to brain damage, depending upon degree of impairment, present a different order of adjustment problems than do seizures and a hemiplegia or seizures and an orthopedic disability. Attitudes—especially those of self-worth, self-esteem and confidence—become differentially exacerbated in the multiply disabled individual with epilepsy.

PSYCHOSOCIAL AND DYNAMIC HISTORY

The mental health clinician should note data about all the above factors as part of the patient's history. Thus, the psychiatric/psychological history, in addition to the usual information and psychological test results (see Chapter 5), should also include a complete history of the patient's epilepsy. The history should be accurate and sufficiently detailed to permit the establishment of:

1. Psychiatric, psychological, characterological-dynamic diagnosis;
2. Behavior associated with the seizure disorder and/or anticonvulsant drugs;
3. Psychosocial adjustment to and coping with seizures and tasks of daily living.

These data should be organized in terms of the patient's developmental stages; at each stage, the neurological, psychological, and social environmental (including ethnic-cultural) reactions to epilepsy should be described in detail covering the areas noted below.

Infancy Through Childhood (birth-5 years)

Neurological History. The patient's age at the onset of seizures is important for determining developmental stresses and arrests, as are the circumstances surrounding the onset. For epilepsy beginning in infancy or early childhood, surrounding circumstances might be febrile, a fall on head, unconsciousness, an infectious disease (for example, measles), breathholding, etc.

The clinician should also note genetic factors, that is, the history of seizures in maternal and paternal family members.

The type of seizures and frequency of occurrence are other important considerations.

Pre-ictal and post-ictal behavior should be described, including such pre-ictal events as an aura, hyperactivity, irritability, or such post-ictal symptoms as confusion, sleep, headache, or muscle cramps. The time duration of each symptom should be ascertained.

The antecedents to seizures should be listed, including any specific sensory, motor, or cognitive/emotional stimuli that trigger seizures, such as hyperventilation or breathholding.

Any sensory-motor deficits, such as numbness or incoordination, should be included, as should cognitive deficits—for example, in number concepts or in memory for nursery rhymes and names.

Other important considerations are the antiepileptic drugs that have been prescribed, their interaction with other drugs, any physical or behavioral side effects, and the degree to which the drugs control seizures (reduce their number over time). The patient's (or, at this age, the parents') compliance to the drug regime is also of paramount importance. The extent of compliance in taking prescribed anticonvulsants should be corroborated by data on drug levels in the blood serum.

Parents and Family. The parents' reaction to the onset of seizure and the diagnosis should be determined. Common reactions include making the rounds—going from doctor to doctor; shock and trauma; acceptance; anxiety; shame and secrecy; overprotection; rejection of their child; denial; or guilt and self-blame.

The therapist should also determine sibling reactions—acceptance, shame, denial, hostility, etc.—and the reactions of other family members, such as grandparents and close relatives: Do they accept or reject the child? Are they critical of the parents or supportive of them vis-à-vis epilepsy?

The parents' general knowledge and understanding of epilepsy and of their child's seizures can influence how they relate to their child. How accurate is their information and how well do they apply this knowledge in the management of their child's seizures and adjustment? Related to this is the parents' involvement with epilepsy, as well as the nature and degree to which epilepsy dominates their lives. Are the parents members of epilepsy self-help programs or voluntary epilepsy organizations in their community?

The Patient. The therapist should note the child's behavior, including evidence of hyperactivity or hypoactivity, withdrawal, clinging to parents, lethargy, depression, retarded or arrested development, or the presence of another behavior problem.

Environmental Reactions. The reaction of other people in the community is significant for the epilepsy patient's adjustment. For the young child, environmental reactions might include the reactions of nursery and kindergarten teachers—acceptance, rejection, undue restrictions; neighbors' reactions—for example, allowing their children to play with the child with epilepsy, exchanging baby-sitting arrangements, or being willing to stay with the child with an epileptic seizure disorder.

Childhood Through Late Childhood (5-11 years)

Neurological History. The neurological history should cover the points noted for the younger child. In addition, the clinician should secure data on cognitive deficits (memory, reading, quantitative ability, concreteness) and perceptual motor development.

Parents and Family. The information on parents and family should include the points noted for the younger child.

The Patient. At this stage, more information can be gained from and about the child him or herself. The child's reaction to the disorder and the seizures is important. Does the child respond with fear, depression, anxiety, relaxation, or what?

The reactions to taking medication should be ascertained. Is the child depressed, resentful, rebellious, noncompliant, or is he or she responsible for and taking his or her own medication? Are there side effects such as depression, drowsiness, hyperactivity, psychomotor retardation, or gingival hyperplasia?

The child's performance in school is also important. The therapist should determine the child's academic standing and any evidence of learning disability. Is he or she is at the proper grade level? In a regular or special school program? The child's interpersonal relations with peers and authority figures should be ascertained.

The child's involvement in community activities, for example, cub scouts, scouts, after-school programs, 4H clubs, or Y programs should be determined.

Environmental Reactions. At this time, acceptance by school administrators and teachers without undue restriction is important as is acceptance by the community, that is, neighbors and clubs.

Any physical and psychological trauma arising out of seizures should be noted—for example, physical injury or being scapegoated by peers (such as being called names).

Early Adolescence through Early Youth (11-19 years)

Neurological History. The neurological history at this time is the same as for earlier developmental levels. In addition, the therapist should ask whether a girl's menstruation is a trigger for seizures, as in catamenial epilepsy.

Parents and Family. Age-specific additions to the history should include the parents' attitude toward independence: permission for driver's education and driving a car (if state license requirements are met); keeping up with a peer group; leaving home for prep and boarding school and college; and choice of vocational careers.

The Patient. At this point, the therapist should explore the patient's sexual feelings and outlets and dating habits. Recreational skills such as social dancing, skiing, tennis, and contact sports become more important, as do interpersonal relationship skills and group participation. Prevocational activity and career choice, including permission for afterschool employment, are significant. Alcohol and drug attitudes and use should be explored. The therapist should elicit the patient's reaction toward growing up and gaining independence.

Environmental Reactions. The therapist should find out whether the patient is permitted participation in high school sports, accepted into college, admitted into a college dormitory, accepted by fraternities and social clubs and by employers. Any imposed restrictions should be noted.

Young Adulthood (21-40 Years)

The Patient. Age-specific additions to history include the patient's attitudes toward seizures—specifically, the extent of self-knowledge and its use in personal management of the disorder. The therapist should note details of the patient's adjustments such as depression, resignation, denial, anxiety, being a shut-in, acceptance and coping.

Also to be noted by the therapist are the patient's attitudes toward travel, public transportation or driving a car; dating, marriage, having a family, and sexual adjustment; having seizures in the presence of one's mate or children, at work or in public; the ability to discuss epilepsy with the mate, and carry out family planning; and community involvement.

Environmental Reactions. Environmental response at this stage consists of the extent to which job and career development are restricted or unrestricted by the seizure disorder; employer acceptance or rejection; availability of life insurance, major medical, and automobile insurance; participation in a company social or sports groups, for example, a bowling league.

Middle and Old Age (40-65+ Years)

The Patient. Age-specific data to be added to history include family attitudes toward seizure patient: acceptance/rejection/overprotection. The patient's attitude toward the life changes that may occur at this time should also be ascertained, for example, living alone and ability to manage seizures, and the ability to travel. The therapist should note the patient's attitudes toward seizures: anxiety, fear, depression, acceptance.

Environmental Response. At this point, employers may wish the patient to take early or forced retirement. The acceptance, rejection, or restrictions placed on the patient by senior citizens' communities, nursing homes, retirement communities are also important.

PSYCHOLOGICAL TESTS

The increased likelihood of the presence of organic signs and cognitive deficits, of psychosocial maladjustment, and of reactions to being on anticonvulsant drug regimes for years in persons with epilepsy,[18,19] justifies the psychological testing of patients before starting psychotherapy. The Neuropsychological Battery of Epilepsy and the Washington Psychosocial Seizure Inventory (described in Chapter 5) were specifically designed to evaluate these functions in patients with epilepsy. Psychotherapeutic interventions benefit from having an accurate profile of these factors for each patient at the start of therapy. They are especially important when devising and implementing the treatment plan. These test batteries—including the traditional tests as the Rorschach, TAT, MMPI, etc.—alert the therapist to such factors and provide an objective measure of the extent of the patient's memory deficit, degree of sustained attention or distractibility, perceptual motor functions, defenses, and personality organization.

For example, H.B., a 31-year-old male with complex partial seizures (psychomotor), complained of poor memory, of having been left out of sports at college, and of generally poor academic performance in college. He failed several courses and had to take an extra year to graduate. He attributed his poor college grades to his being a "playboy," not studying, and to his lack of interest in books. He showed marked feelings of inadequacy, calling himself "dumb" despite his apparent above-average intelligence.

Psychotherapists experienced in working with seizure patients would clinically assess this patient as having a cognitive deficit manifested by a low attention span and a poor memory, and as having difficulty in reading (dyslexia); they would view his being left out of sports like basketball as probably due to a perceptual-motor deficit which made tasks involving eye-hand coordination difficult, resulting in poor scoring. They would also assess that these complaints are consistent with the organicity associated with a seizure disorder and are not psychologically determined. Having these clinical impressions confirmed by psychological tests not only corroborates the therapist's clinical judgment but enables him or her to use the "hard" objective data to confront the patient without running the risk of the patient's resistance-denial negating the clinical findings. Accepting the assessment is the first step in corrective therapy to help the patient work through his or her feelings of inferiority and rejection.

EDUCATION, COUNSELING, AND PSYCHOTHERAPY

A complete history of the psychiatric, psychological, and social factors related to the individual's epilepsy also makes possible the formulation of a goal-directed treatment/counseling plan directed at enabling the seizure patient to live with maximum independence and actualize his or her potential. This plan would prescribe the nature of counseling and/or treatment of choice to overcome the psychological and social problems interfering with coping and adjustment.

Educational Counseling

Misinformation, myth, and superstition are still rampant among persons with epilepsy and their families, as well as the general public. In some ethnic and cultural groups, seizures are still considered a demonic possession or punishment for some sin. This contributes to the notion of shame and stigma which is still attached to epilepsy.[20] Consequently, knowledge about epilepsy is vital for the patient and the family. The Commission for the Control of Epilepsy and Its Consequences states:

> A concern for knowledge and understanding about epilepsy is necessary from the very first individual with whom the patient becomes involved, whether it is the GP or the internist. All patients want to know what the condition will do to them or their families. They do not understand what is happening to them and they require direct answers to avoid fear of the unknown.[21]

Specific information based on the patient's needs should be given in understandable and usable form to the patient and the family. The information and educational materials should take into account the patient's ethnic background, history, concerns, anxieties, and psychological and social orientation. Periodic updating and reinforcement of knowledge should be included in the counseling program.

However informative printed materials, films, and lectures may be, they still require the patient to abstract and apply the information to his or her own problems—a most difficult task. Nor are these materials usually sufficient to overcome deep emotional sets. These methods cannot, therefore, be used to replace face-to-face educational counseling. Such counseling should be part of the clinical services in every seizure clinic and in the office of every epilepsy specialist. It also should be made available as a patient service, separate and apart from public education, by community health programs such as those of community mental health centers and the Epilepsy Foundation of America and its local chapters.

A clinical example will illustrate the need for educational counseling and its importance. J.K., a 36-year-old machinery salesman, came for general information about epilepsy so that he "could better understand the subject." A brief history disclosed he had generalized seizures (grand mal) which were not completely controlled. It was further disclosed that he had a great fear of having a seizure while on a sales call. He would, therefore, "pop" a Dilantin into his mouth on his way to each customer. On some days he would more than double his prescribed dose and become toxic, reacting with dizziness and ataxia.

Through educational counseling, the client became aware that his "popping" Dilantin did not have the immediate effect of warding off a feared seizure because of the drug's slow action. Instead, the drug overdose made him appear drunk. The educational counseling gave the patient knowledge about the way the anticonvulsant medicines work. It did not, however, eliminate his acute anxiety about having a seizure at work. Accordingly, he was referred for short-term psychotherapy to help him cope with his fear of having a seizure.

Counseling

Counseling addresses the reactive problems arising out of the events of daily living. It is therefore directed at problem solving and the development of skills for coping and adjustment.

M.B., a 28-year-old legal secretary, was referred to counseling because of frequent job turnover despite her excellent skills. The interview disclosed that she had complex partial seizures (temporal lobe epilepsy) of brief duration during which she became incontinent and wet her clothes, the chair she sat on, and the carpet under it. When she recovered from the brief seizure, she became intensely ashamed and immediately left her job without stopping to collect the salary due her. Nor would she return to the job when her employer requested her to. In the reality-oriented (problem solving) counseling, a solution was jointly arrived at by the client and counselor: that the patient wear elastic-rubber incontinent pants and keep a bath towel, soap, and a deodorant in her desk drawer. Thus, after a seizure occurred, she could go to the ladies room, dispose of the urine which had been held in the watertight pants, clean herself, and then return to her desk.

Psychotherapy

The literature, Feldman and Ricks[22] assert, rarely demonstrates a reduction of seizure as a result of psychotherapy. My own psychotherapeutic experience indicates that reduction in seizures which has occurred has most often been the result of the patient's improved drug compliance or his/her changing physicians—that is, to a physician who has a special interest in epilepsy—rather than the direct result of psychotherapy.

I have also found that psychotherapy can result in a marked improvement in patients' acceptance of their seizure disorders, a reduction in confusion, depression, and tension, improved self-esteem and self-confidence, and a greater ability to cope with seizures and the problems they cause in daily living.

Dynamically oriented psychotherapy is the therapy of choice to deal with the unconscious emotional conflicts, deep-seated anxieties and feelings, attitudes, and behaviors which make up character defenses and life styles. Seizures assault ego functioning, causing the individual to respond with severe emotional upset, low self-esteem, and high dependency; in such cases, the individual may require a psychoanalytically oriented therapy, preferably short term.

Persons with epilepsy experience the same anxiety, stress and adjustment problems as do others who require psychotherapy. But because these problems may be caused or exacerbated by their seizure disorder, psychotherapy with the seizure patient calls for a special focus on and consideration of seizures.

While no special analytic procedures are necessary to treat the patient with epilepsy, it is *essential* that the therapist have a thorough knowledge of epilepsy and its neurological, neurobiological, and psychological and social bases—that is, the links in the behavior chain and their role in the individual's maladjustment.

Dynamic Short-term Psychotherapy

For seizure patients, an effective dynamically oriented short-term therapy program is the therapy of choice. According to Wolberg, there are definite operations in such a program.[23] These operations, modified to accommodate them to the problems of patients with seizures, are discussed in the sections which follow.

Establish a Positive Working Relationship (A Therapeutic Alliance)

A climate of warmth, understanding, and acceptance is a prerequisite for achieving a positive working relationship. Empathy is a particularly indispensable personality quality that helps to bond a good therapeutic alliance. A therapist who cannot accurately feel what it is like to have seizures and the experiences they provoke is apt to convey a detached professional attitude to the seizure patient. This will militate against developing a working, therapeutic relationship essential if therapy is to proceed. In addition, verbalizing the patient's feeling about seizures when he or she is unable to do so and reassuring the patient that his or her situation is not hopeless also strengthen the therapeutic alliance.

Deal With Initial Resistance

Too often the seizure patient has been so disappointed by helping professionals that he or she may defend against having his or her hopes raised. This may be manifested in a lack of motivation. If constructive therapy is to follow, then this source of resistance needs to be recognized and neutralized.

Take the History

In addition to the usual psychological diagnostic history, it is essential to record the patient's feelings about seizures, take note of the anticonvulsant drugs used and any side effects (see pages 34-40), and obtain the psychometric test data (see Chapter 5). Details of the seizure may require interviewing family members. If the patient is given colored crayons and paper and asked to draw his or her seizure state while talking about the drawing, one can often obtain the subjective emotional representation of the seizure for the patient. The data from this initial interview should enable the therapist to establish the etiology or psychogenic bases and to formulate a tentative psychosocial diagnosis and psychodynamic description.

Define the Precipitating Events

The events directly responsible for the patient's present upset or why he or she has come to psychotherapy at this time should be defined, as should the role, if any, of the epilepsy as a precipitating factor in the patient's current behavior.

Formulate a Dynamic Picture Which Explains the Patient's Behavior

The dynamic picture of behavior may be defined first from the patient's past and present history, appearance, attitudes and reactions, including those to the therapist and to the treatment situation in general. Unconscious materials such as dreams and fantasies, associations and non-verbal signs also help in formulating the dynamic assessment.

This formulation, in simple, clear, direct descriptive-explanatory sentences, should be given to the patient after the initial diagnostic interview. This gives the patient a coherent picture—a cognitive map which links past and present behavior, the role of seizures, and how he or she has learned his or her adaptational life style. This will help explain the precipitating factors in the context of the individual's seizure disorder, previous experience and history, and personality structure.

The dynamic explanation of what is going on with the patient, given in language and concepts which the patient understands, will help to dissipate the confusion which is common in nearly all persons with epilepsy. Such an explanation offers the patient hope for change and is in itself an effective motivator for therapy to proceed.

Make a Tentative Psychological Diagnosis

A descriptive psychosocial diagnosis stated in behavioral terms may help circumvent the difficulties of the current psychiatric nosology and at the same time serve as a basis for selecting the treatment plan of choice to achieve the stated therapeutic goal. Additionally, this type of diagnosis will prevent persons with epilepsy from being classified as having fixed characteristics (often labeled "*the epileptic personality*"). The diagnosis will also provide data for research into the adaptational patterns which correlate with seizures and their consequences.

Select a Focus for Therapy

The therapist chooses the symptoms, behavioral difficulties, or conflicts which clinical judgment indicates are most amenable to change. These may include depression resulting from uncontrolled seizures, inability to gain employer acceptance and thus employment, or anxiety and tension associated with the fear that others will learn of the patient's epilepsy, leading to social rejection.

The patient's active participation in the selection of the therapeutic focus and goals, and in the therapeutic process, is essential for the successful outcome of the therapeutic alliance. This is especially important for the patient with epilepsy who has learned to passively follow physician's orders and hope that the problem will automatically be ameliorated. It is, therefore, necessary to explain to the patient in specific terms his or her *active* role in goal setting and in the psychotherapeutic process. This shared approach will offset the seizure patient's usual passive role in therapy and gain the required active participation.

A verbal contract that spells out the patient's active role, the time and frequency of appointments, the number of sessions, and the termination date will solidify this arrangement.

Goal setting by patients correlates with positive psychotherapeutic outcome. The total number of sessions should be limited—about 20—yet be sufficient to achieve a limited goal. The low number avoids reinforcing dependency—a characteristic common to persons with chronic disorders such as epilepsy. By so doing, the therapist joins with the seizure patient's deep, and often unexpressed, striving for independence.

Select Therapeutic Techniques

Epilepsy requires a therapist to be active and flexible in applying a range of techniques that will carry out the treatment plan and that are acceptable to the patient. The techniques include supportive, educational and psychoanalytically oriented interventions, psychotropic drugs, hypnosis, biofeedback, behavior therapy, individual, group, couples and family therapy, and any combinations of these in order to help the patient with his or her immediate problems as revealed by the diagnostic history.

Use Reactions and Defense Patterns Revealed in Therapy

Any intervention designed to change behavior patterns associated with seizures will bring out the patient's defenses and resistances. Identifying these patterns of defense and resistance and interpreting them to the patient in a compassionate way can be a deeply felt revelation. The resulting insight, while alone insufficient to produce change, can be used by the patient with the aid of the therapist to learn new adjustment patterns to replace maladaptive ones.

Focus on Present

Although present-day adjustment patterns have their origins in past relationships with parents, siblings, and other significant people in development, nevertheless the therapeutic focus is on the here and now reactions to epilepsy and its consequences. When a patient shows an awareness of or makes a connection with the past, this should be acknowledged by the therapist. But in keeping with the time frame of short-term therapy, delving into the past is not encouraged.

Accept Positive Transference Reactions

The warm, nonjudgmental, accepting therapist encourages the patient with seizures to exhibit positive feelings and attitudes toward him or her as an idealized authority figure. These feelings are accepted without interpretation, for they foster a reduction in tension and support the placebo element that promotes therapeutic change.[24] Negative transference reactions, on the other hand, must be dealt with rapidly and with empathy lest they impair or break the therapeutic alliance.

Watch for Countertransference Feelings

The person with epilepsy may evoke in the therapist frustration, anger, irritability, boredom, dislike, or extraordinary interest. These feelings on the part of the therapist, if they continue without his or her personal examination, may interfere with a good working relationship and impair the therapist's objectivity. The reactions, however, can be used in the service of therapy, for they alert the therapist to the possibility that the patient's behavior elicits similar reactions from others.

Beware of Resistance

However much an individual's reaction patterns to his or her seizures may be self-defeating, they are familiar and constitute a known equilibrium. Any change calls forth a counterreaction to maintain the status quo so as to hold on to the secondary gains of epilepsy. This resistance, which often exists outside the patient's awareness, needs to be openly shown and interpreted in a non-condemning manner.

Assign Homework

The patient should be asked to keep a diary recording problems with seizures; conditions and environmental stimuli which precede seizures; and new responses to the epilepsy in general and to seizures in particular. Following a learning paradigm, the patient should be instructed to catch him or herself when responding to epilepsy or seizures in an old way, and to take an action which uses a new response based on newly gained insight and understanding.

When the patient successfully uses the new response, he or she should be instructed to note it and to reward him or herself for it (see Figure 1). Thus, the patient can learn new ways to reverse destructive adjustment reactions to epilepsy and seizures, and *actively* use them to achieve the desired change in behavior.

Set a Termination Date

As the termination date approaches, remind the patient so that it is fixed in his or her mind. Separation anxiety and negative transference are usual at this phase of therapy, and a possible triggering of seizures may occur. These should be interpreted as they arise. The seizure patient's dependency and fear of autonomy, as well as the comfort in continuing therapy, may be present without his or her awareness.

On the termination date, to avoid the feeling that the patient is being

FIGURE 1

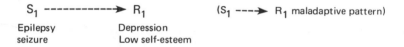

Observe or catch the old, maladaptive response (S_1 ---→ R_1) pattern and use this insight; think of a new adaptive response (R_2) to (S_1) and use it for change.

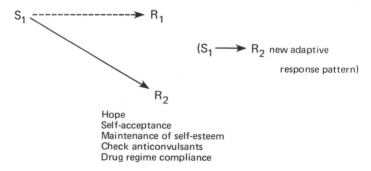

The new response R_2 needs to be reinforced by rehearsal and self-rewards. This will help extinguish the old maladaptive pattern.

abandoned by the therapist, suggest that the patient write you about his or her progress from time to time.

Use Post-therapy Assignments

The chronicity of seizures and their consequences makes a continuing vigil of primary importance, lest the newly gained behavior patterns be eroded under the battering of seizures and environmental forces. The patient must be alerted to this possibility and shown how to deal with it. Accordingly, persons with seizures must also be educated as to the signals of regression so that they can take active steps to remedy environmental factors that can be changed while at the same time accepting the irremedial ones—including the seizures themselves.

Further Treatment

For some seizure patients, the severity of the seizures and the lack of support from family and environmental systems make long-term supportive therapy necessary to maintain their homeostasis. Peer groups offer this type of support network. Other patients who have shown little improvement with the short-term therapy approach may need long-term reconstructive therapy.

Other dynamic therapies that are useful for reconstructive personality and behavior pattern change and which can be used either conjointly with individual therapy or separately are discussed below.

Provide a Referral to a Helping Resource

Referral is a therapeutic operation that is essential for the seizure patient, who is often beset by a multitude of problems ranging from the social and economic to the abridgment of basic human rights. Many of these problems require recreation and social groups, housing, employment, or advocacy and legal action for their solution. Thus, it is necessary to seek the intervention of social, health, and welfare agencies with expertise and resources to address these issues on behalf of the person with epilepsy (see Chapter 9 for resources).

OTHER DYNAMIC THERAPIES

Group Therapy

Analytic group psychotherapy is a useful approach that can be used to correct distortions which affect interpersonal relationships. It is particularly applicable to the seizure patient, who is beset by these problems. The group should consist of eight to ten patients, with varying types of psychopathology, age, gender, lifestyle, and defenses. Groups composed solely of persons with epilepsy are likely to limit reconstructive efforts. The similarity of these patients' experiences and perceptions due to seizures, the communality of their defenses, and the individual resistance to change may join to form a group resistance. A heterogenous group which includes two or three members with epilepsy (to prevent the person with epilepsy from feeling different or isolated) and others who do not have epilepsy is preferred. The group therapy modality can provide the seizure patient with a corrective emotional and behavioral experience, especially as the transference distortions are worked through.

Couples Therapy

Interrelations between the couple themselves and between the couple and other people are addressed in couples therapy. The distortions, problems, and difficulties arising out of or complicated by the seizure disorder in one or both members are brought to the awareness of the couple and worked through in the therapy.

For example, E. and B.F., a couple married 17 years with three children, came to therapy because of marital difficulties. The man was 40, the woman 38. Mutual sets of interlocking guilt were uncovered. His guilt stemmed from his obsessive effort to control his uncontrolled temporal lobe epilepsy (complex partial seizures) and his feelings of not being perfect and manly because of them; this increased his dependency. Her guilt came from the belief that she was responsible for his seizures. She attributed her emotional outbursts and impatience as the triggers for his attacks. Her guilt at the thought of leaving her husband with his uncontrolled seizures and dependency prevented her from seeking a divorce, and this exacerbated her conflict. Couples therapy enabled husband and wife to gain awareness of and understand their respective difficulties, specifically the role epilepsy played in their marital problems. The therapy reduced their fighting and enabled each of them to see that some of their problems stemmed from deeply rooted individual psychopathology, which was triggered by the epilepsy, and not caused by it.

Family Therapy

The interrelations in the family, between the nuclear family and the extended family, and between the family and the community at large—friends, neighbors, church groups, etc.—and the way that these interactions and interrelationships are affected by the presence of a seizure disorder in a family member often make family therapy the desired method of psychotherapeutic intervention. This therapy permits the family members to ventilate their feelings about epilepsy, get the catharsis, and then work through their feelings and restructure them. The change in feelings and attitudes among the various family members often results in a relief of anxiety, tension, depression, resentment, etc., which can do much to restore homeostasis in the family. When the family member with epilepsy is a child or adolescent, such intervention can also prevent pathological psychosocial adaptation from developing.

Eclectic Therapy

The varied presenting problems that a person with epilepsy brings to a therapist often require the application of a number of complementary and adjunctive therapeutic procedures. The self-regulatory (relaxation) therapies may reduce fear and anxiety associated with having a seizure; behavioral therapy, in combination with anticonvulsant drugs, may help reduce or control seizures. Behavioral methods include desensitization, to prevent a specific sensory antecedent from triggering seizures; aversive conditioning, to neutralize specific motor antecedents such as hand-waving or eye-closing from setting off a seizure; and biofeedback to promote relaxation and possible control of seizures (see Chapter 2).

These therapies or any combination of them are used to obtain symptom relief and varying degrees of personality restructuring.

CONCLUSIONS

The psychodynamic therapist has a significant role in the psychosocial management of the patient with epilepsy. Specifically, it is to provide an understanding based on all the factors arising out of the patient's epilepsy and its impact on adjustment to independent living and to use this assessment to formulate a treatment plan. Often the plan will require that the dynamically oriented psychotherapist orchestrate a strategy which will sequentially call on the specific counseling and other therapies to address the multifaceted presenting problems.

For example, a patient who is confused and depressed by uncontrolled seizures and who has little accurate knowledge about epilepsy needs educational counseling, neurological management and possibly neuroleptic drugs. If after an appropriate trial on anticonvulsant drugs seizures persist, then adjunctive behavioral therapies such as biofeedback, conditioning and hypnosis should be explored. For a patient whose memory deficits are symptomatic of the seizure disorder and not of mental retardation, remedial educational counseling would be used to find cognitive avenues for helping retain items in memory. The patient would also require counseling to accept his or her memory deficit as a result of a neuronal condition, without assaulting him or herself for stupidity. Such acceptance will be ego enhancing and prevent the erosion of self-esteem and confidence.

An individual who has been made dependent by seizures or by parents' attitudes toward them can benefit from analytic reconstructive therapy to change his or her traditional mode of responding to epilepsy (defensive character armor or lifestyle), and to nurture and release independence. So does the individual whose narcissism requires seeing each seizure as a sign of not being perfect and as a narcissistic injury, thus denying them to the point of nonacceptance of the diagnosis and noncompliance with the anticonvulsant regime. Individuals who have been so traumatized by rejection—real or fantasized—as a consequence of their seizures that they become withdrawn and socially isolated also require dynamic psychotherapy, particularly conjoint individual and group therapy.

It is only through the judicious use of all therapies and counseling, self-help groups, and other aids available through effective information, referral, and advocacy programs (see Chapter 9), and after a careful diagnostic assessment of the psychosocial adjustment problems, that the individual with epilepsy can approach an actualization of abilities and capacities consistent with his or her interests. It is only then that the person with epilepsy can be released from assaulting anxiety, depressions, stress, and feelings of low self-worth to achieve self-fulfillment.

REFERENCES

1. Lennox, W. G. *Epilepsy and Related Disorders.* Boston: Little, Brown & Company, 1960.
2. Williams, D. T., Gold, A. P., Shrout, P., Shaffer, D., and Adams, D. The impact of psychiatric intervention on patients with uncontrolled seizures. *J. Nerv. Ment. Dis.* 167:626-31, 1979.
3. Feldman, R. G. and Ricks, N. L. Nonpharmacologic and behavioral methods, 89-111. In: Ferriss, G. S. (ed.), *Treatment of Epilepsy Today.* Oradell, N.J.: Medical Economics Co., Book Division, 1978.
4. Ibid.
5. Wolberg, L. R. Handbook of Short-term Therapy. New York: Thieme-Stratton, Inc., 1980.
6. Commission in *Plan for Nationwide Action on Epilepsy.* The Commission for the Control of Epilepsy and Its Consequences, Vol. II, Part 2, p. 358, U.S. Dept. of Health, Education and Welfare, DHEW Publication No. (NIH) 78-276, 1978.
7. Arangio, T. A Position Paper: A Systemic Examination of the Psychosocial Needs of Patients with Epilepsy: The Need for a Comprehensive Change-Approach. Commission for the Control of Epilepsy and Its Consequences, Vol. II, Part 1, p. 376. U.S. Department of Health, Education, and Welfare, Public Health Service, National Institute of Health, DHEW, Publication No. (NIH) 78-276, 1978.

8. Wolberg, L. R. Psychotherapy and the Behavioral Sciences. New York: Grune & Stratton, 1966, pp. 62-64.
8a. O'Leary, D. S., Seidenberg, M., Berent, S., and Boll T. J. Effects of age of onset of tonic-clonic seizures on neuropsychological performance in children. *Epilepsia* 22:197-204, 1981.
9. Herrmann, B. P., Schwartz, M. S., Karnes, W. E., and Vahdat, P. Psychopathology in epilepsy: Relationship of seizure type to age at onset. *Epilepsia* 21:15-23, 1980.
10. Lennox, 1960, op. cit.
11. Pond, D. A. and Bidwell, B. H. A survey of epilepsy in fourteen general practices. II. Social and psychological aspects. *Epilepsia* 1:285-299, 1960.
12. Sands, H. and Price, J. C. A pattern analysis of the Weschler-Bellvue adult intelligence scale in epilepsy, Vol. XXVI. *Epilepsy*, Proceedings Association for Research in Nervous and Mental Disease. Baltimore: The Williams & Wilkins Company, 1947, pp. 604-615.
13. Feldman and Ricks, 1978, op. cit.
14. Ibid.
15. Ibid.
16. Ibid.
17. Lennox, 1960, op. cit.
18. Dodrill, C. B. A neuropsychological battery for epilepsy. *Epilepsia* 19:611-623, 1978.
19. Dodrill, C. B., Batzel, L. W., Queisser, H. R., and Temkin, N. An objective method for the assessment of psychological and social problems among epileptics. *Epilepsia* 21:123-135, 1980.
20. Jilek, W. G. The epileptic's outcast role and its background: A contribution to the social psychiatry of seizure disorders. *J. of Operational Psychiatry* 10:127-133, 1979.
21. Commission, 1978, op. cit.
22. Feldman and Ricks, 1978, op. cit.
23. Wolberg, 1980, op. cit.
24. Ibid.

7

THE CHILD WITH EPILEPSY: PSYCHOTHERAPY AND COUNSELING

ROBERT G. ZIEGLER, M.D.

Childhood epilepsy is not an uncommon problem. Perhaps 90 percent of all epilepsy patients experience their initial seizure before they are 20 years old. In order to treat some of the common problems which children and their parents may experience in relation to epilepsy, the various forms of childhood seizures should be understood.

The three most common periods in which epilepsy appears are the first 2 years of life, the ages between 5 and 7, and the early years of puberty. The incidence and type of seizure are often related to age of onset (see Figure 1).

Infantile spasms (see page 16) usually begin between the ages of 3 and 24 months.[1] With the onset of the spasms, development may slow down or regress. The prognosis is gloomy, and mental retardation is often an accompaniment. There is some evidence that there is a better prognosis in idiopathic cases than those in which there is an underlying disorder,[2] although in all cases of convulsions of the newborn, parental reactions require understanding and counsel.

Absence attacks (see pages 14-15) may begin between the ages of 3 and 12. These seizures often disappear by the age of 20. Medical treatment is most successful, and there are not as many psychological complications.

Major motor (grand mal) epilepsy is frequently encountered in children. Witnessing these attacks may be frightening to parents, and this type of epilepsy can have extensive ramifications in the family system.

Partial complex (temporal lobe) seizures (see page 00) may have unusual presentations in childhood. Children often have trouble describing these attacks and may merely appear frightened and run to the mother. Parents may overlook motor features and complain only that the child is unresponsive

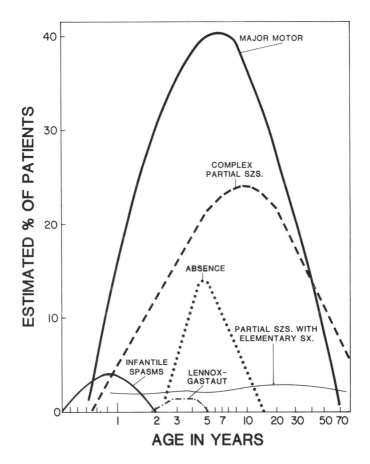

Figure 1. Incidence and type of seizure related to age

at times. This form of epilepsy is often associated with behavioral problems, such as hyperkinetic activity, that can be severe. The temper outbursts and poorly controlled behavior may be a greater handicap than the seizures themselves. In the older age group, varied bizarre motor or psychic experiences may be found associated with this type of epilepsy in adults (see Chapter 3). The diagnosis, treatment, and personality impact of these seizures are complex.

The combination of absences, atonic/tonic attacks, and myoclonic seizures (see pages 16-17) is often medically difficult to treat. The "drop" attacks may be very disturbing for parents, since the child suddenly sinks to the ground.

There are often associated retardation or learning dysfunctions, psychomotor slowing, or other signs of central nervous system dysfunction.

The seriousness and long-term effect of various seizures on a patient's adaptive efforts are still a matter of some debate. Data regarding the specific outcome of different seizure patterns and their interaction with other factors affecting adjustment are incomplete. Whitehouse's study of 200 children presenting at John Hopkins' Seizure Clinic compared these patients to a standard sample and a group of controls from a cerebral palsy group. The study concluded:

> It would appear that children with seizure disorders show a wide range of cerebral dysfunction with mental retardation at one end and no detectable dysfunction at the other end. The occasional existence of retardation is no new fact, but these results emphasize the existence of a considerable number of children with either milder retardation or, more importantly, cerebral processing problems such as is seen with minimal brain dysfunction.[3]

Harrison and Taylor's 25-year follow-up study of epilepsy presents additional worrisome evidence. One in every 10 children died within the 25-year span. Among the surviving population, slightly more than one in 10 were permanently confined to institutions. A little more than one-fifth of the sample had chronic epilepsy.

Different epilepsies are associated with different dimensions of ictal (seizure) and inter-ictal (between-seizure) disturbances. The impact of a particular seizure disorder depends on its symptomatic or clinical expression and its interaction with the life stage of the child and family when it occurs. Seizure disorders also create a fluctuating impairment. The frequency and type of seizures may change. Prior to a seizure, a child may be irritable as in the prodrome of other illnesses. The specific psychological impact of seizures on children and families results from repetitive, *unpredictable* electrical discharges that can disrupt any ongoing activity and the social context within which it occurs.[5] The developmental lines of autonomy (sense of *control* of self and social context) and competence (sense of *mastery* of external environment) are particularly prone to impairment in epileptic children. These difficulties can be exacerbated by the family's fears and instinctive reactions to overprotect or ignore. Thus, the context within which a youngster masters control of self and environment can be constricted or fraught with anxiety.

PSYCHIATRIC/PSYCHOLOGICAL DIAGNOSIS

The mental health practitioner seeing a youngster with epilepsy should obtain from the child's neurologist or pediatrician an understanding of the nature of the seizure disorder, the frequency with which the seizures occur, current medication and its behavioral side effects, any known prognostic leanings, and a rough estimate of the contribution of the neurological disorder to current behavioral or symptomatic picture. In addition to this information, the clinician needs a working framework in which to place the data.

A Diagnostic Model

To plan an effective psychotherapeutic intervention for the child and his or her family, a thorough diagnosis must be implemented in order to evaluate a confusing array of variables. In a child with a seizure disorder and a "behavioral" or "psychiatric" problem, the nature of the difficulty may lie in the manner in which the seizure disorder affects the adaptive abilities of the child or the system that contains him or her. The major systems within which the child operates are home, school, and peer group; all have a feedback effect on the child.

A diagnostic model should provide a tool to consider the developmental stage of the child, the specific organic impact of the neurological disorder (or fluctuating electrical disturbance), and the current nature of the systems within which the child functions, as well as their interrelationship. At distinct points in time, manifestations of the child's evolving cognitive and affective organization (stranger anxiety or separation protest, for example)[6] result both from neurological maturation and from experiences that are acquired and stored through repetitive interactions with other systems, each with its own brand of organization, point in a life cycle, and demands.

The cybernetic model stresses that the behavior of any part (individual child) of a system (such as family, school, or peer group) may be understood in terms of the *present* organization, functioning, and interaction of that system. Behavioral changes are seen as the result of positive feedback or negative feedback effects.[7,8] Feedback flows in two directions. The child may introduce disequilibration into a surrounding system by the nature of his or her behavior (feedback). The child's state elicits a reaction (fear, concern, anger) which may then shape new behavior which is directed to him or her. The limitation of the cybernetic model, with its emphasis on open systems in which all interacting components may be seen in fluid equilibrium, is in regard to those variables (pieces of behavior or internal organization) that may have a fixed basis, as well as those that have a higher than expectable threshold of change.

Neurologic dysfunction may produce behaviors which, while appearing to be in dynamic equilibrium with an external system, continue unmodified even with shifts in the organization of the external system. A good diagnostic evaluation should define the symptoms most likely to change through intervention.[9]

Another point of organization to be considered is the relationship between one action and "the relations which it bears to other processes."[10] Adaptive functioning concerns not just correct pieces, but those pieces in combination with the proper timing.

An error may occur at one or many points within a system. A diagnostic model must be broad enough to help tease out these parts. This is crucial in dealing with the neurological organization/dysfunction, self and system interface, since a seizure disorder could, for example, introduce an error of timing. In order to plan a treatment strategy to offset this problem, the location in the system of the error needs to be specified as accurately as possible. Is it within the central nervous system, within one of the systems that provides the adaptive context, or between them?

Compensations for errors can occur naturally or can be fostered by interventions. Once the point of the error has been defined, one can consider how to develop a correction, either from within (CNS), without (systems), or through prompting a new relationship between the two. This complex task confronts us when we wish to foster the adaptive abilities of an epileptic child. Diagnosis must suggest the point of vulnerability in order to plan the best intervention.

Geschwind emphasizes the necessity of resolving this diagnostic dilemma with neurologically based disorders. "Organic lesions can lead to changes in behavior, which in many instances are uninfluenced by the past experience of the animal. . . . Hence, the strategy of 'looking at the whole patient,' which is often so useful to the psychiatrist in other circumstances, may be actively misleading when certain discharging or destructive lesions of the brain are present."[11] When diagnostic assessment suggests that we cannot necessarily expect change in the primary symptom, we must then try to make sure that negative feedback cycles do not exacerbate the problem. Additionally, we can attempt to create positive feedback cycles that may either diminish the frequency of the symptom or fail to reinforce it.

The diagnostic dilemma posed by epileptic children is underlined by Whitehouse, who states, "Learning disabilities may produce behavior problems and behavior problems may interfere with learning and both may reflect underlying dysfunction in the nervous system."[12] Within these confusing circular reactions, the diagnostic model suggested here defines the different points of possible impact of dysfunction. The impact of dysfunction must be separately assessed in each aspect of the system. For instance, decreased attentiveness of a youngster may create a strong negative feedback effect within a school environment, while it could be less crucial at home. Or one aspect of a child's functioning could have an impact on another internal component: Impaired attentiveness on the part of the child exerts greater effects on a child's overall performance when there are associated impairments in cognitive abilities.

The three functions that require diagnostic assessment in a youngster with seizures are: 1. attention and engagement (attention is closely tied to engagement, a psychological state of interest and connectedness which affects a youngster's involvement with different objects, situations, and people); 2. cognitive style (analytic or impulsive, particular tactics of understanding) and cognitive abilities (IQ, academic levels, particular areas of competence); and 3. affective states, including perception, expression, how the child feels he or she is understood by others, and how the child recognizes the affective states and expressions of others.

Each of these three central areas of functioning should, of course, be considered within the limits of the child's general developmental stage. Each should also be appraised in the different settings within which a child functions. Crossover effects between systems can be noted, for example, when a youngster's bad morning at home affects school performance, or when a youngster's difficulties with peers leads to a decline in a parent's esteem. Just as internal parameters can affect functioning in different settings, each system can operate in such a way that the child's functioning is markedly different.

The Family

As noted above, the family is one of the major systems in which the child operates. This section will discuss diagnostic considerations concerning the family.

The Impact of Chronic Illness. From a psychiatric viewpoint, the onset and course of any chronic medical illness has some predictable impact on the family. A chronically ill child may become the focus of family attention as well as the perceived (and, in fact, real) culprit for disturbing the family homeostasis. Chronic illness—depending upon its severity—may alter many household routines and demand new ones. The most disruptive diseases are those which demand total involvement. The worse the prognosis, the greater the stress is on the family.

A family is more able to be supportive to a child when he or she has already developed a personality and/or has been previously healthy. The earlier the onset of the disorder, the greater the possibility of parental guilt feelings. The more burdensome the child becomes, the greater the possibility of resentment, projected blame, and ready disappointments. Often the defense for many of these affects and worries is denial. Denial, while at times an effective mechanism, can inhibit the family's ability to create flexible accommodations to the child's impairments.

In chronic medical illnesses of children, mourning is an ongoing phenomenon.[13] At each developmental stage, there is probably one reminder or another of a youngster's deficits or differences in comparison with other children. Attendant to this, the child's ability to "contribute," a source of maintaining family cohesion, is impaired. In the absence of this role for a child, the parental response of frustration and resentment can grow, as can the child's sense of loss and low self-esteem. Each child needs to have a positive place in the family despite the limitations imposed by an illness.

In addition to accepting the sadness of an ongoing loss, the child and the family must be able to tolerate the "elemental destructiveness" of the child's illness, as well as the child's primitive fury at himself, his parents, and his own body. The parents need to be able to contain and survive the anger they experience in order to hear and heal the child's anger.

In brain-injured children, the additional complexity of neurologically determined lability, irritability, and impulsivity[14] can further impede the family's task of helping the child deal with anger. The family's sense of being trapped or isolated with this child, as well as the often real desertion of extended family members, heightens the difficulty in discriminating between the child's easy anger and frustration secondary to his or her limitations (those times when the child needs supportive understanding) and the impulsivity and aggression evoked by central nervous system irritability and easily triggered by external stimuli (when the child needs clear and uniform limits). In order to help parents accomplish the difficult task of differentiation, diagnostic understanding must be constantly updated to take into account the child's and family's evolving life tasks, the neurological disorder, and the child's overall developmental state.

In addition, there are likely to be family problems specifically associated with epilepsy. For example, Ward and Bower state, "One can predict that either severity or frequency of seizures above a certain level will be likely to precipitate social and management problems, either in the patient or the family."[15] Parental fears that Ward and Bower document as associated with epilepsy include a realistic fear of injury, fears of "mental abnormality" (including retardation, personality change, behavioral irregularities), fear of social handicaps, and fears about etiology, drug treatments, and future handicaps.

The Family Diagnostic Interview. When working with children, one of the best ways to get an initial reading of a problem is to have a family interview. Skill in dealing with families is as essential to effective work with an epileptic youngster as knowledge of the whole body is to the doctor who treats the child's neurologic problem. Family sessions allow one to begin to deal with the guilt, anger, and denial reaction and to define the manner in which the system operates, positively and negatively, in regard to the "identified illness." One of the benefits for those working with neurological disorders is that we can attribute "the problem" (however it has been defined in our referral) to the youngster's medical situation. One of the comforting initial statements that can be used is, "Seizure disorders place a burden on both parents and children; by talking together, we can often better understand how the seizures have affected your youngster and the entire family. We can then work out the best possible way that your doctor and others can be of help." This kind of statement tends to reduce most families' reflex guilt reaction and allows them some relief, even when the youngster's problem is secondary to the underlying family pathology.[16] The "identified illness" can also be the starting point for requesting other changes in the family system.

The initial family interview permits an assessment of the quality of parental sympathy and understanding of the youngster's disorder. The family life stage and the parents' personality styles can be defined. Is the family overburdened, either by the demands of the reality of the illness or family members' own feelings of guilt and anger? Different channels of communication within the family can be surveyed: 1. parent-child, 2. mother-father, 3. husband-wife, and 4. sibling-sibling. The family's organization should be considered. The recent suggestions of Tseng and McDermott[17] on family classification provide a quick overview of the parameters of assessment that should be considered, including the family life stage, the marital relationship, the parent-child subsystem, the nature of the organization of the family group, and the degree of connectedness between the family and external supports and their interaction.

Having a good opening line does not assure, however, that all family members will be cheerfully lined up outside your office. In some instances, where the family is somewhat chaotic or has multiple subsystems, you may see different bits of the family accompanying the child to different sessions. With some adolescents, it is worthwhile to begin to discuss their situation with them *before* discussing their situation with the family. Where there is overt denial, however, it is often best to begin with a group interview. As in one's approach to most clinical problems with children, a comprehensive guideline to organize the collected data can allow much flexibility in interviewing patterns.

In the initial diagnostic interview, one of the most commonly sounded themes has to do with the parents' sense of guilt, or, as it is suggested derivatively, their lack of trust in their parenting. ("Are we doing the right things?" "Have we created this?" "Have we made it worse?") Parents' hopes for the "right" way of parenting leading to a "cure" need to be addressed immediately in order to assure a less confrontational interview ("You're the expert! Tell us what to do") and a better clinical alliance. Helping parents understand that you know that the usual complex task of parenting is compounded by a seizure disorder and its effects often leads to audible sighs of relief. At the same time, however, the point of the interview—to understand, perhaps to find a way to make things easier by working together—must be stressed so as not to contribute to the chronically underlying wish that it will all get better and/or just go away.

There are some common dilemmas in the subsystems of the epilepsy patient's family. Parents, siblings, grandparents, and extended family are prone to some particular failings. As can be readily imagined, parents are most vulnerable to their guilt and anger. Apart from the particular effect of these feelings on the behavior of a mother or a father, the seizure disorder of the child often splits the parents along two common dimensions: limit setting and involvement. Typically, the mother polarizes to overprotective overinvolvement and non-limit setting, and the father towards harshness and distance. These differences can further increase any underlying marital split. The grandparental generation often has a tendency to side with one point of view or the other. This further inhibits the possibility of some modulated combination of limit setting and involvement. Grandparents sometimes step into a primary caretaking role and thus further undermine the parents' sense of trust in themselves. Normal siblings often react with a lot of anger, about which they experience guilt, and may then either be drawn into a reactive parental role or withdraw silently, reducing the patient's chances for some direct feedback. The extended family often simply deserts. Their awkwardness in the face of the youngster's illness and their fears of what might be asked of them prompts distance that isolates the family with the ill child.

The Tools for Family Assessment. During the first interview, it is useful to develop a three-generational diagram (Figure 2) to convey a sense of the family system of origin of each of the parents, other important supports or relationships, and the existence of other concomitant problems or medical disorders. The diagram creates a framework within which one can quickly

ILLUSTRATIVE THREE GENERATIONAL GENOGRAM

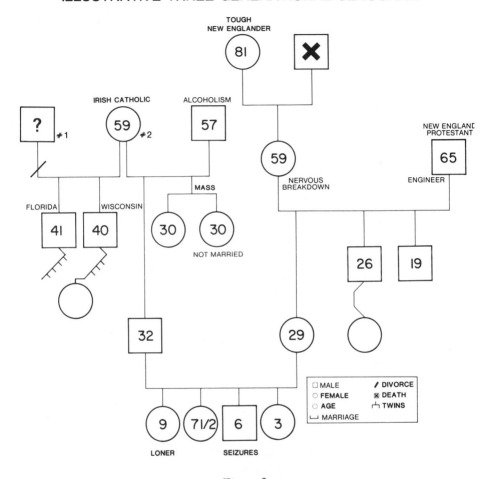

Figure 2

check out possible parental power conflicts (for example, eldest married), compatibilities (for example, oldest brother from one family married to youngest sister in another), bases for identifications with the patient, or other significant aspects in the family history (ethnic conflicts, parental loss of parent in early life, other family members' illnesses, or "black sheep" siblings).

The family session permits one to observe those behavioral sequences which have a repetitive character. They may be suggestive of an underlying family rule which defines how the family maintains homeostasis.[18] For instance, if a family has difficulty with anger about the illness and this topic is touched upon, one might find that one member's understanding may be quickly followed by another's denial while a third begins a disruptive tactic. All of the general diagnostic expertise which one brings normally to family interviews[19,20] is just as important where a particular member suffers from epilepsy.

The Child

In each era of childhood, different affective states are defined and integrated with the youngster's view of him- or herself and his or her world. Without adequate synthesis, denied and defended affects can begin to distort a youngster's functioning, world view, and interaction with others. Children also need to begin to learn the impact of their emotions and behavior on others and how to interpret and deal with other people's expressions and actions.

The preschool child presents him- or herself as an immediate and direct amalgamation of the various forces that contribute to his or her state at a particular moment: temperament,[21] current state of cognitive development,[22,23] overall exposure to and interest in life,[24] and family situation and security. All of these currents flow together, combine with characteristics of stimuli in the present moment of meeting, and reveal themselves. In regard to the preschool child with epilepsy, one is more likely to see the effects of a cognitive delay, the possible impact of a post-ictal state, the effect of medication, the possibility of hyperactivity, or an anxious reaction primarily determined by parental management rather than the particular youngster's worry or reaction to having epilepsy.

Once a child reaches school age, the ability to reflect on his or her own state and condition is more evident. The child can define his or her worries and notice if he or she is different. In this age group, once again, the primary reaction does not appear to be having epilepsy. Youngsters seem quite able to endure the occasional seizure. When seizures are difficult to control and the youngster needs to wear a helmet or have activities circumscribed, other reactions do appear. School-age children react more to other overt aspects of their possible brain damage: if there are associated learning dysfunctions, for example, or if another physical handicap is present. Conversely, the child can be the object of central nervous system dysfunction when it creates background irritability, decreased attentiveness, or hyperactivity. The "why me?" reaction begins at about age eight or nine. Some youngsters may also have a transient reaction to taking medication at school, especially if the seizure disorder begins in the midst of a youngster's school career. The greatest number of complaints in this age group arise from those consequences of epilepsy which make one different: the medication routine, the occasional attack, doctor's visits, and so on. The reflection of a family's worries and fears, its sense of the child as damaged, may also begin to affect the image the youngster has of him- or herself, even if there are no other associated disabilities.

Some of the more serious psychological complications of epilepsy begin in early adolescence and extend into young adulthood. Many of the consequences of the long-term interactions, flowing from the family system's way of managing the fact of epilepsy in the child's life, begin to develop. The *family* two main developmental lines of the adolescent in which difficulties occur are autonomy and competence. When the family has had a constricted, overprotective attitude, adolescent rebellion and negativism can set in. If the family has attempted to adopt an offhanded denial of the problems, youngsters may react with even more denial and begin to refuse their medications and disregard some sensible precautionary warnings. The early adolescent is ready to demonstrate autonomy ("I can do it myself!") and competence ("I can do anything!") in their most extreme forms.

The growing awareness of self and others that occurs in adolescence affects youngsters with epilepsy in many ways. They have an increased sensitivity to taking or carrying medicine. The issue of a driver's license begins to loom large. In most states, the driver's license is contingent upon the patient having a doctor's note saying the patient has been seizure-free for at least 18 months. This may be difficult since, during puberty, there may have been a transient increase in the frequency of seizures.

Post-ictal states and transient seizures make teenagers vulnerable to attack for being "dopey," "crazy," or "off-base" by their peers and/or teachers. Longstanding learning dysfunctions and their characterological consequences[25] may also become more apparent. For the adolescent who has had only rare seizures and therefore has maintained a low profile as far as epilepsy is concerned, the beginning intimacies between boyfriend and girlfriend may bring feelings about having epilepsy to the fore. Questions regarding marijuana, alcohol, drugs, and sexual feelings may complicate adolescents' attempts to sort out feelings about themselves and the world.

Depending upon the degree of compromise in adaptive (social, learning, and psychological) behaviors that coexist with epilepsy, questions regarding the overall competence of the adolescent begin to be faced. In earlier years, these could be put off by child and family—awaiting maturation, new medication, or a stroke of luck. Now they become prominent. The frequency of epileptic seizures, for example, has serious implications with regard to the job market, quite apart from the stigma that is so often attached to listing "epilepsy" on job application forms. Feelings about the adolescent's ability to live independently away from home become important. Each of these questions, as well as their associated realities, has serious consequences for the adolescent's view of himself and the world.

The Child's Diagnostic Interview. The basic tools the diagnostician brings to the interview with the child are his or her knowledge and personality. The ideal therapist is a relaxed, open, and inquisitive person who is able to connect to people, whatever their background and life stage, with language and imagery[26] appropriate to them. The therapist is able to listen and to detect from the shared information the point at which a particular person or family system may be vulnerable, as well as the complex connections that the vulnerability may have to social and psychological defensive structures, other beliefs, and adaptations. From the very first, however, the therapist must communicate an attitude summarized by the Greek word *agape*—"a disinterested, objective, willing of the best for a person regardless of how one feels toward him."[27] The willingness to help, understand, and to care enough to expect the best effort of the patient and family in difficult and painful situations cannot be replaced. The ability of the therapist must make it possible to interview a family and consider the painful dilemma that both parents and children may be struggling with from very different and often disharmonious points of view.

In the interview with a child, the therapist's language needs to be adjusted to the level of the child. Questions and information that the child may find helpful must be interpreted (for example, "I know that when Mommy and Daddy cry, you sometimes feel scared"). Communication with a child is often facilitated by play. Play, in the diagnostic interview, may serve two purposes (besides providing the context for multiple observations): 1. the nature of play can be viewed as communication in itself, the metaphor for the dilemma of the child; or 2. play can be the comforting background (like coffee and doughnuts for adults) within which an adult and child communicate seriously about the child's thoughts, observations, and worries.

Drawing, as a part of a play interview, provides an avenue for cognitive and projective assessment. During the initial interview with a child, it is often valuable to ask the child to draw a person, draw his or her family, and draw his or her family doing something. The child's approach to the paper, his or her sequencing in drawing, and the associated memories this task can evoke are often helpful in developing a picture of the child as a person.

The Tools for Child Assessment. Since epilepsy is a symptom emanating from the central nervous system, it is important to be able to assess the child from a cognitive, organic point of view. Planning and help for a child with seizures must include a sense of the youngster's cognitive style, ability to learn, and ability to attend and engage. The possible impact of learning dysfunctions, hyperactivity, and the effects and side effects of medication on children with seizures must be remembered. Medication can depress a youngster's functioning as well as contribute to a picture of hyperactivity.[28]

It must also be considered that electrical discharges in the brain, even if not strong enough to prompt a full-blown seizure, can affect behavior. Just as we know that the prodrome of illness in children or the existence of fever can cause behavioral irregularities and dysfunction, we also must consider and learn more about the behavioral and cognitive impact of subthreshold seizure discharges on states of affect, attention, and cognitive processes.

Psychological testing of cognitive functioning and academic achievement are often invaluable aspects of a youngster's diagnostic assessment. The sophistication of the instruments and the level of complexity of the neuro-psychological testing has a great range (see Chapter 5). It is best to start with simple IQ testing. For youngsters below the age range of the WISC-R, the McCarthy Scales of Children's Abilities is a useful instrument. During the play interview, an easily administered task is Bender-Gestalt cards.[29] Astute clinical observation of how children solve different tasks and problems within the play interview and in the structured testing situation, added to academic achievement tests, will indicate whether discrepancies suggest that more sophisticated testing is needed.

It must be kept in mind that office examinations, including the pediatric neurological, the play interview, and psychological testing, are poor indicators of hyperactivity, since the structure, low level of stimulation, and one-to-one situation all contribute to reduce hyperactive behavior. An attentional disorder must be considered as an aspect of the diagnostic assessment whenever the presenting picture of a youngster includes a majority of the following: decreased attention, increased activity, decreased achievement, increased anger and aggressiveness, decreased peer associations, and labile affect. One of the easiest ways to do this is through the use of one of the rating scales from the Hyperkinesis Index,* which is based on a questionnaire developed by C. Keith Connors (see Figures 3 and 4).

Throughout the play and family interviews of the child, one can monitor the parameters of attention/engagement, cognitive style, and awareness of internal affective state and its impact on others. Each of these factors can be compromised in an epileptic youngster. The degree and nature of the

---

*The Index is not a valid instrument for diagnostic purposes. At present no norms have been established for the questionnaires; therefore, it is not possible to determine the degree of abnormality represented by any given score or range of scores on the questionnaires.

Teacher's Questionnaire

Name of Child _____   **Grade** _____

Date of Evaluation _____

Please answer all questions. Beside *each* item, indicate the degree
of the problem by a check mark (✔)

	Not at all	Just a little	Pretty much	Very much
1. Restless in the "squirmy" sense.				
2. Makes inappropriate noises when he shouldn't.				
3. Demands must be met immediately.				
4. Acts "smart" (impudent or sassy).				
5. Temper outbursts and unpredictable behavior.				
6. Overly sensitive to criticism.				
7. Distractibility or attention span a problem.				
8. Disturbs other children.				
9. Daydreams.				
10. Pouts and sulks.				
11. Mood changes quickly and drastically.				
12. Quarrelsome.				
13. Submissive attitude toward authority.				
14. Restless, always "up and on the go."				
15. Excitable, impulsive.				
16. Excessive demands for teacher's attention.				
17. Appears to be unaccepted by group.				
18. Appears to be easily led by other children.				
19. No sense of fair play.				
20. Appears to lack leadership.				
21. Fails to finish things that he starts.				
22. Childish and immature.				
23. Denies mistakes or blames others.				
24. Does not get along well with other children.				
25. Uncooperative with classmates.				
26. Easily frustrated in efforts.				
27. Uncooperative with teacher.				
28. Difficulty in learning.				

Figure 3. In each of these rating scales, there are ten items correlated with hyperactivity /attentional deficit syndrome. Each of these items is scored from 0 (not at all) to 3 (very much). Thus, a score can range from 0 to 30. Scores over 15 should increase one's concern about this possible diagnosis. The key items in Fig. 3 (Teacher's Questionnaire) are 1, 3, 7, 11, 14, 15, 16, 22, 26, & 28. The key items in Fig. 4 (Parent's Questionnaire) are 4, 10, 11, 13, 19, 25, 30, 31, 33, and 37. (Distributed by Abbott Laboratories, North Chicago, IL 60064)

Parent's Questionnaire

Name of Child   **Date**

Please answer all questions. Beside *each* item below, indicate the degree of the problem by a check mark (✔)

	Not at all	Just a little	Pretty much	Very much
1. Picks at things (nails, fingers, hair, clothing).				
2. Sassy to grown-ups.				
3. Problems with making or keeping friends.				
4. Excitable, impulsive.				
5. Wants to run things.				
6. Sucks or chews (thumb; clothing; blankets).				
7. Cries easily or often.				
8. Carries a chip on his shoulder.				
9. Daydreams.				
10. Difficulty in learning.				
11. Restless in the "squirmy" sense.				
12. Fearful (of new situations; new people or places; going to school).				
13. Restless, always up and on the go.				
14. Destructive.				
15. Tells lies or stories that aren't true.				
16. Shy.				
17. Gets into more trouble than others same age.				
18. Speaks differently from others same age (baby talk; stuttering; hard to understand).				
19. Denies mistakes or blames others.				
20. Quarrelsome.				
21. Pouts and sulks.				
22. Steals.				
23. Disobedient or obeys but resentfully.				
24. Worries more than others (about being alone; illness or death).				
25. Fails to finish things.				
26. Feelings easily hurt.				
27. Bullies others.				
28. Unable to stop a repetitive activity.				
29. Cruel.				
30. Childish or immature (wants help he shouldn't need; clings; needs constant reassurance).				
31. Distractibility or attention span a problem.				
32. Headaches.				
33. Mood changes quickly and drastically.				
34. Doesn't like or doesn't follow rules or restrictions.				
35. Fights constantly.				
36. Doesn't get along well with brothers or sisters.				
37. Easily frustrated in efforts.				
38. Disturbs other children.				
39. Basically an unhappy child.				
40. Problems with eating (poor appetite; up between bites).				
41. Stomach aches.				
42. Problems with sleep (can't fall asleep; up too early; up in the night).				
43. Other aches and pains.				
44. Vomiting or nausea.				
45. Feels cheated in family circle.				
46. Boasts and brags.				
47. Lets self be pushed around.				
48. Bowel problems (frequently loose; irregular habits; constipation).				

Figure 4. In each of these rating scales, there are ten items correlated with hyperactivity /attentional deficit syndrome. Each of these items is scored from 0 (not at all) to 3 (very much). Thus, a score can range from 0-30. Scores over 15 should increase one's concern about this possible diagnosis. The key items in Fig. 3 (Teacher's Questionnaire) are 1, 3, 7, 11, 14, 15, 16, 22, 26, & 28. The key items in Fig. 4 (Parent's Questionnaire) are 4, 10, 11, 13, 19, 25, 30, 31, 33, and 37. (Distributed by Abbott Laboratories, North Chicago, IL 60064)

compromise affect the treatment plan. When attentional capacities are diminished but engagement with the environment is intact, medication or environmental change which expands the youngster's ability to attend can create a marked improvement. Where engagement is also diminished, motivating the youngster and reattaching him or her to an enriching and consistent environment are doubly necessary. If a youngster's cognitive style consists of two parts rigidity and one part denial, initial environmental changes and psychotherapy may be necessary to increase his or her flexibility. Where a youngster has a poor awareness of internal states or of their impact on others, the parents, school, and therapist can often mount a triple approach to heighten a youngster's internal and external social awareness.

The Problem List

Once family and child assessments have been made, the mental health clinician must establish whether or not there is a problem. A problem list must also be generated from four points of view:

1. What is the problem from the point of view of the referring agent (e.g., uncooperative or complaining patient)?
2. What is the problem as seen by the parents (e.g., child has seizures)?
3. What is the problem of the child (e.g., don't know)?
4. What is the problem as seen by the mental health professional (e.g., chaotic, multi-problem family)?

The parenthetical remarks suggest that problem definition can at least define quickly the degree of trouble one can expect in working with a particular situation!

The task that remains for the mental health worker is how to reconcile the presenting problem with the difficulties as he or she has assessed them. Sometimes this may be difficult to do. However, the information that has been gathered may be of use to the child and family through other avenues. The assessment can influence plans and approaches taken by other systems that provide the family's medical care, the child's schooling, or other social supports.

In generating the problem list, asking different family members to keep a log of different behavioral baselines is very useful. In addition to providing a parameter upon which to gauge the impact of one's intervention, this task can interrupt troublesome or escalating behavioral sequences. Furthermore, behavioral logs have the effect of heightening the child's and family's awareness of the child's behavior and its interactional setting. Often some sympathy and distance on the part of the family members can be obtained.

Therapeutic Interventions

Once a problem has been defined, there are many forms of intervention that can be considered. In the long-term care of the seizure-disordered patient and family, different approaches may be useful at different points in time. Some of the more common forms of treatment and their application to different aspects of seizure-related problems will be reviewed in this section.

Play Therapy

Play therapy is a useful modality for the anxious, constricted child or one who has a particular confusion in regard to his or her view of self, illness, or family's reactions. Play interviews can create a sound basis for work and rapport with families and parents.

If the child's anxiety is associated with specific areas of inhibition, it is well to combine play therapy with a clear definition of the problem areas in order to monitor whether there are gradually increasing behavioral repertoires. In many cases, one must be aware that parental anxiety about the child's seizures leads to the definition of "dangerous" play. During the diagnostic phase, one must be careful to separate these two phenomena.

For the anxious epileptic child under five, a therapeutic nursery school program with parent support and education groups is the best alternative to play therapy.

Parental Counseling

During the preschool and early school-age period, counseling is often necessary for the parents of epileptic children. Common fears, a sense of embarrassment or guilt, failure of limit setting ("It's so terrible that he has epilepsy, how can we always be reprimanding him?"), or overprotectiveness are all avenues of exploration in counseling. Some of the most common secondary psychological complications in epileptic children are the result of untreated parental anxieties which become embedded in the family system.

Family Therapy

Family therapy is often best used during the early adolescent and adolescent era. Often, the mutually exclusive systems of denial (Parents: "I can't let him do that"; Child: "Epilepsy doesn't stop me from doing anything") need conjoint attention before other, more individualized forms of treatment can be defined. Common concerns about epilepsy affect issues of competence and autonomy in both the family and the adolescent.

Group Therapy

Group therapy is a treatment that can approach problems associated with epilepsy with diverse formats for reality testing and peer interaction. Apart from seizure clinics, however, there is not always a large enough population of epilepsy patients to be served by group treatment. Within seizure units, groups may be useful for parents of children with particular syndromes (for example, Lennox-Gastaut) or parents of children who have just been diagnosed. During early adulthood, when issues of employment may be a serious concern, programs such as the Training and Placement Service created by the Massachusetts Epilepsy Society make use of a wide variety of support groups, role-playing groups, and task-centered groups. For the adult population in many areas, epilepsy information groups that meet on a monthly basis with invited speakers often play an important role for continuing education and support.

Casework Interventions

It should be remembered that finding out that one has a chronically ill child is an extraordinarily disorganizing event. Parents, no matter what their socioeconomic status and educational background, need clear information (see Chapter 9) about state assistance programs for disabled children, where medical and social service care is most available, routes to obtain a second medical opinion (often a phase associated with coming to terms with a diagnosis of epilepsy), and whether special education or other programs may be needed for their child. These casework interventions are often excellent ways to do derivative counseling based on the multiple issues that arise in dealing with an epileptic disorder.[30]

Task-Focused Interventions

For many people, "psychological counseling" is still anathema. One must remember that this obstacle can be overcome by selecting a task to do together. Where both parents and child are particularly worried about the child's functioning, carefully selected and graduated tasks that the parents can help the child accomplish are a great substitute for talking about worries! Instead, one talks about how to get the job done with the least stress for all concerned.[31]

Behavioral Therapies

The application of behavioral therapies to the treatment of seizures has been discussed in Chapter 2 and in the epilepsy literature.[32] These therapies can also be applied to the treatment of "psychological" symptoms. Often, accomplishing the specific reduction of a particular symptom is therapy enough for some children and their parents. In other cases, it is just one necessary component of an overall treatment plan.

Where it is possible to reduce symptomatology, one has an *obligation* to do so. Any decrease of disturbing behavior on the part of children reaps rewards for the child and the entire family. Behavioral guidelines and techniques of behavior modification and management should be part of the repertoire of skills of any therapist who treats children and does school consultation. Sometimes it is too easy to forget that removing symptomatic behavior is as important as understanding it. The experience of seeing an entire family system look different through the reduction of stress which was prompted by a troublesome behavior is the best way to learn this lesson.

Medication

The diminution of symptomatic behavior is an important goal in the use of medication as either ancillary or primary treatment. The diagnosis and treatment of hyperactive, aggressive, or attentionally deficient behaviors is a key factor in the care of the child with seizures. Many of these youngsters have associated brain damage and, thus, a higher incidence of a "hyperactivity," "MBD," or the attentional deficit syndrome. It should be remembered that the symptomatic picture may not be brought to the therapist's attention until adolescence. Stimulant medication, along with seizure medication, still has an important role. The guidelines for the medication treatment of adolescent and adult disorders of anxiety and depression follows that of other psychiatric populations.[33] This holds true for the use of phenothiazines for a psychotic disorder associated with seizures, although consultation with the treating neurologist is imperative.

Alternative Uses of Therapists

There are a number of families, children, and adults with whom a psychotherapeutic contract cannot really be fashioned. In a number of these cases, the referring problem is the patient's failure to comply with one aspect or another of good medical and self care. In these instances, one can delineate how some of these problems may interlock with other defenses and investigate what way the neurologist can best handle the person's failure. Many times, it is possible to say, "You are here only because you failed to do X; I am sure that I can convince your doctor that you needn't come to counseling if you take care of this." Put bluntly, the trip to the psychotherapist is a threat and can be used as a behavioral inducement for the patient to take better care of him- or herself. For some patients and families, it is easier to comply with the neurologist's requirements than to subject themselves to counseling. For those who are more ambivalent, more choice can be allowed the family, for instance: "I'd really love to meet with you all, but if you do X and Y, there really won't be a problem left, will there?"

Systems and Network Interventions

In many families, long-term assistance is best mobilized through other systems that can be of support to the child and family. School consultation is often a key factor of assistance. When special programs are needed, it should be remembered that their primary objective is not to cure seizures, but to assist problems of learning dysfunctions, decrease hyperactivity, or remediate other developmental delays. Like parents, school personnel often need information about the nature of seizures and reasonable guidelines for management of the attack and post-ictal states. While this information may be brief, it can often take over two hours just to elicit and listen to people's fears so that the basic guidelines can be understood comfortably. Like parents, too, school personnel may need repeated reviews. Schools should not succumb to the cloak of secrecy. Teachers should be encouraged to have small discussion groups and share information with the student peers when appropriate. Audiovisual aids are also available.

The family with an epileptic child often winds up being isolated from members of the extended family. Network mobilization[34] and educational meetings with various members of the extended family are often invaluable aids. The extended family can offer added information, peer counseling, and an exchange of points of view, as well as providing possibilities for respite care.

As children grow up, more supports may be necessary, in serious cases, to allow them to begin to function independently as young adults. Knowledge of halfway houses, cooperative residences, and community training and employment workshops thus may be a vital part of a family intervention.

Crisis Intervention

Many families are not willing or able to make a long-term, or even a short-term, therapeutic contract. In these cases, the particular vulnerability and needs of a family and child should be documented during crisis interventions. These sporadic contacts, at times of crisis, can help maintain and support the family's healthy aspects and attempt to derail malignant, negative feedback cycles. The basic understanding of the family should be communicated to the medical care agent, school systems, and other agencies which may have a continuing role or involvement with the family.

CASE EXAMPLES

The focus of my work at the Seizure Unit has been to understand and help ameliorate the developmental challenge presented by epileptic attacks to the child and family. My interest in the two developmental lines of autonomy and competence in children and their interaction with family systems has led to many questions related to a youngster's cognitive functioning and associated affective experiences. The flow, pattern, and mechanisms of exchange within different family systems and the developing child with seizures were accentuated. The case histories presented here point to different vulnerabilities that may emerge along the developmental course of child and family.

The Infant with Seizures

The infant with seizures presents the parents with the problems associated with an impaired child, leading to the inevitable reactions of shock, denial, a sense of loss and shame, questions of guilt and blame, anger, and recurrent periods of depression. For example, one mother is quoted as saying, "I find it very hard not to be angry at the world. The doctors say that if my baby could have been treated even a week or two sooner, he might not be so badly retarded. We tried, but we couldn't seem to find any doctor who understood it was epilepsy until it was too late."[35]

While this quotation suggests many of these elements of a parent's reaction, it also raises questions in regard to complications of medical management (see below). These complex reactions on the part of the parents also set the stage for the compromises which can occur in the development lines of autonomy and competence in the child.

The Preschool Child with Seizures

Kenny was 2½ years old when a mixed seizure disorder (atypical absences, grand mal, and atonic attacks) began. The year following the diagnosis was a difficult time for all. Kenny's seizures were hard to control, and his parents vacillated between hopes for a cure, denial, depression, chaotic over-concern, extreme anxiety, and moments of calm acceptance. By the time Kenny was 4¼, some of these concerns became further complicated by his short attention span, hyperactivity, difficulty in modulating aggressivity (associated with parental confusion), and clear signs of developmental delays: poor motor coordination, poor articulation, and visual motor problems. The parents' concerns were exacerbated by the excitement Kenny created in a half-day nursery program by both his behavior and seizures. The teachers also told the parents of his difficulties with age-appropriate activities.

Here, in addition to much parental counseling and medical backup, early educational intervention and a wide array of supportive services needed to be defined for this youngster. Frequent school consultations, to allay the anxieties of the teachers and to help educate them about guidelines for seizure management, could decrease the chance that Kenny would be further ostracized and isolated. Clear support was necessary for parent and child to allow Kenny to function away from his mother's care so that he could consolidate a better sense of autonomy. The long-term process of modifying his educational environment to support his ability to be competent was only beginning.

The School-age Child with Seizures

A mother brought her son Richie, aged 8.6 years, to the local emergency room after the boy had a seizure while on his bicycle. The boy had a black eye and required stitches on his forehead. As a result of the concern in the emergency room at the local hospital, the boy was transferred to Children's Hospital. By the time the doctor saw the mother at Children's, she was very upset. She was crying and complaining about the medical care Richie received. She said, "The doctors tell you to try and treat him normally, let him be an active boy, but then when they see him bleeding they stitch him up and rush him to the hospital. They act like I did something wrong. Should I feel bad about the bruises? I called the doctor the other day and told him I was worried and he said, 'Yes, yes, come in for your regular appointment at the clinic.' Now they tell me Richie has to be admitted to the hospital."

Treading the fine line of "normalcy" can be difficult for everyone involved. One of the important issues to be aware of in treating seizure disorders is the fine balance of denial and acknowledgment required in order to deal with epilepsy. In a sense, epileptic children and their families need to have the ability to cross the street while still watching out for cars, neither huddled together on the street corner nor impulsively darting into the road. This balance is difficult to maintain in managing children with epilepsy, for the guidelines tend to shift. Parents need a great deal of support from those who work with them in order to maintain some degree of flexibility.

The general clinical management of the school-age child with seizures is well defined by Voeller and Rothenberg.[36] They suggest that parents' and children's attitudes about the illness may significantly influence the therapeutic course, within "predictable patterns which form a recurrent theme during the diagnostic and therapeutic phases of management." Their article stresses careful attention to the group of patients whose seizures are relatively well controlled and whose prognosis is good.

Three of their most salient points follow. The first is to clarify what the patient or parents believe the terms "epilepsy," "convulsions," or "seizures" mean and to encourage the patient (child or adult) and family to describe their emotional responses to the seizure. Mental health professionals can clarify the relation between a family's style and the risks inherent in their way of managing a child with seizures. The understanding of the particular vulnerabilities in either parent, the child, or the family system which the seizure disorder may evoke can lead to the most efficient long-term management plan.

Second, Voeller and Rothenberg state, "Parents have remarkably varied and naive fantasies regarding the causality of seizures." There may also be many fears which develop around the concept of "brain damage," especially since, for many people, the distinctions between "craziness," "nerves," and "brain abnormalities" are quite hazy. You need to know what people's ideas are before you begin a process of reeducation.

Third, many of the problems during the long-term care of epilepsy may be related to Voeller and Rothenberg's "FAGS Syndrome"—their eponym for Fear, Anger, Guilt, and Sadness. They believe this syndrome appears to be present to some extent in all cases of epilepsy. For instance, when a mental health worker knows that there have been pressured requests for a new medication regimen, evaluation for surgery, and so on in a case that is relatively benign, counseling often needs to focus on how "sad it is to know a youngster has been saddled with this extra problem to deal with." The other aspect to consider here is that during the initial phase of accepting a child's illness, parents often strike a bargain with the doctor, as follows: "If we follow your orders and try as hard as we can, our child will be cured." When this bargain does not pay off, there is often a renewed flurry of consultations, investigations, and, soon, a search for a new "bargain."

The School-age Child with Seizures and Hyperactivity

Epilepsy is one of the few chronic medical illnesses associated with a higher incidence of hyperactivity.[37] Therefore, in the presentation of a behavioral or academic difficulty in a youngster with epilepsy, the additional diagnosis of an attentional deficit disorder, with or without hyperactivity, must be considered.

Charlie, aged 9.2 years, was referred by his teacher for overt aggressiveness toward his peers. He had well-controlled absences. His greatest difficulty occurred during the unstructured period of the day. Although described as a very verbal child, he had difficulty resolving conflicts with his peers. The Connors Scales that teachers and parents filled out resulted in high scores. During the family interview, it was discovered that the father, reared in Switzerland and now a successful businessman, had been placed by his mother in a children's home for a year and a half because of his overactivity and difficulty in modulating his aggression at age six. Charlie's difficulties were further exacerbated by the fact that his high verbal abilities allowed him to define his ill-timed behavior but did not give him the ability to restrain it. This increased his sense of frustration and sadness, which made him more apt to lose his temper. Stimulant medication plus a focused intervention for Charlie, some help for the parents on management skills, and school consultation were required.

School-Age Children with Seizures and Learning Dysfunction

Mark, an 11-year-old boy, was referred for evaluation because of his poor temper control and associated depression. In addition to his seizure disorder, he had a learning disability (he was in an appropriate class) and was quite awkward. However, in spite of his bad temper, he was a nice kid. The treatment agenda included work with him on a model to focus on his learning difficulty. This project would challenge his patience, expose his difficulty with following instructions, and highlight some of his troubles with coordination.

Mark loved cars and liked building auto models. Model building had been a source of much difficulty in the home, since his younger brother liked models and did them with ease. While working on a model would be stressful for Mark, it would provide an opportunity to review many issues and see how his feelings and reactions led to further trouble for him.

In the course of our model building, however, I learned something I did not expect. We had spent a couple of sessions working on the engine and then mounting it on the chassis. At one point Mark declared, "Let's leave those out," referring to two plastic gizmos that went somewhere alongside the engine. Since he was in charge (and we had had enough struggles that day anyway), I silently assented to his definitive command. Later that month, he was finished assembling the body of the car and was ready to put the two pieces together. He left that day before doing so, and I tried it when he was gone. There was a very poor fit. During the next two or three days, I wanted to sneak back to the Unit while he wasn't there and fix the parts so that when we worked on the model, things would be "easier" and would "look better." There I was, debating a behind-the-scenes patch-up job, when I knew how many hours I had spent unraveling the complications resulting from various families' patterns of "helpfully distorting" the feedback that they gave their epileptic children.

The point of this anecdote is to highlight what a powerful stimulus a youngster's chronic illness can exert upon involved caretakers. The most striking impact of these *distortions of feedback* is on the child's development of a sense of autonomy and competence. These distortions in feedback can be relatively consistent over long periods of time and can therefore exert a powerful effect.

For instance, many youngsters with seizure disorders have a delay in visual-motor skills. They may have trouble reproducing a flower or a three-dimensional square, doing a Draw-a-Person test, or with the Bender-Gestalt cards. During the tasks, they will often remark, "That's no good," "I don't draw too well," "It never comes out right," or "I don't like doing this stuff." We must remember that children—with and without learning dysfunctions—are in the process of creating some complex cognitive categories. Just as a youngster of two or three codifies and labels a large number of different configurations as "house," so does a youngster of five or six begin to have a notion of "what people drawn by six-year-olds look like." Therefore, when we tell the child it's not so bad, or act in a reflexly reassuring manner, it is useless. The youngster is right. He or she must accept this trouble as part of him- or herself. Youngsters are continually acting, estimating, and reacting. Their sense of competence is fashioned from multiple experiences.

The Adolescent with Seizures

A concerned middle-class family came for their appointment at the Seizure Clinic following their 17-year-old son's recent increase in psychomotor (complex partial) epileptic attacks. Both mother and father were present. As the doctor asked about Don's current status, the mother described the number and type of attacks he had had. She kept in close contact with his school so that she was also very aware of any seizures he had there. (While a question of overinvolvement should be checked, those extra tasks are often vital for the child's care and the life of the family. However, it can prompt a certain distortion in family life.)

The father maintained a "concerned silence" throughout the interview and was manifestly anxious when the doctor asked him for his opinion. He had many fears of having to "manage" his son. When the doctor asked if anything was different recently, the mother described how her son had been sleeping less, smoking more, and had recently watched a TV program late at night about a racing car driver which had gotten him very excited and involved. Don's seizures were frequent enough to prevent him from getting a learner's permit. As the mother's description proceeded, Don began to look glum and resentful and sank lower in his seat. When the doctor asked him what he felt, Don refused to answer.

In a separate interview, Don bitterly described how he felt that his parents would always say that what he did—if they disapproved of it, especially—caused more seizures. Now he felt his mother did not want him watching television late at night. She would always say, "You need your rest." They would argue if he drank coffee, went out for a hike, or listened to records late at night. The mother and father both felt that if Don behaved "right," his seizures would not be so frequent.

The constriction in an adolescent's sense of autonomy and competence is often associated with compensatory familial protectiveness. Each nourishes the other. This cycle needs to be teased apart bit by bit. Medical personnel may address this concern from time to time, but painstaking family treatment, associated with specific tasks for family and individual, is often needed to break apart a long-standing adaptation.

Often the specific positions or rationalizations adopted by both individual and family indicate the need for some medical reeducation in order to allow therapeutic restructuring of the situation. If this medical support is available, conjoint examination of the evolution of the constricted field of operation of both the individual and family is easier.

In this painful process, the therapist acts as an emotional container (see Winnicott's notion[38] of the holding environment of the parent) for the fears of death and pain that the family has experienced. Although the therapist supports both individual and family while restructuring aspects of the family, permission for the adolescent to explore new adaptations must be granted.

Malignant Intrafamilial Spiral

Crises often occur in early adulthood when the patient leaves high school and faces the question of functioning independently away from the family. In the absence of some degree of success, retreat from the world can occur in which the patient tries to carve out a bit of control within the family.

A 36-year-old woman who had lived at home since her successful completion of an A.A. degree at a community college was repeatedly turned down in her job applications because she had epilepsy. The family believed she had lost her confidence and never regained her courage. Since she had been at home, she had gone out less and less, and for the past eight years had tyrannized her parents. She turned off their television at night and tucked the parents in so that they would be "well-rested." She had tantrums if her parents went somewhere she did not like; consequently, to avoid conflict, the parents stayed home more and more.

Her brother reported that their mother and father no longer permitted the patient to go out alone, and she had taken over the household. The parents had become increasingly fearful that the patient would fall or have a seizure; whenever she was asked to do something at home, she would have a tantrum or a seizure.

The stage for this psychologic familial disorder was set in early childhood by the parents' fears. The brother reported that their father always said that the patient would not live long and that they had to make her happy. Whenever she didn't like her supper, the father would take her out to a restaurant. The mother would spend hours fixing the patient's hair so that it would be "just right." In spite of these continuing interactions and others, the patient was quite outgoing and successful at school. In the absence of alternative activities, however, she gradually focused her attention on managing her home life and that of her parents.

Here, the issues of control and autonomy have been negotiated within the context of the seizure disorder itself. The seizures can become a way in which a child—rarely granted control—can gain control of the familial environment. The disease becomes the child's competence, rather than a limitation. This autonomous capture of control can represent a real, although problematic, achievement by the epileptic individual, and a continuing perplexity in the life of the family.

This complex adaptation—the use of seizures as a means of gaining control—suggests why one often sees patients who have both "true" and "false" seizures (see page 22). The seizure disorder, the act itself, has become an ingredient in the modulation of internal states or external adaptations in the interpersonal and social environment. These adaptations and their function are often difficult to clarify. Often this difficulty is a reflection of the fact that the patient has never made a "crisp" adaptation in the first place, and there are numerous concurrent muddles.

MEDICAL MANAGEMENT: FACILITATOR AND COMPLICATOR

There are different sorts of vulnerabilities that can be defined under different medical conditions. Briefly, four of them are (1) the expert syndrome, (2) the chronic illness/acute doctor syndrome, (3) the misunderstanding/anger complex, and (4) the iatrogenic consequences of hope.

In the expert syndrome—where the family finally arrives at the specialist's doorstep after having seen many other doctors—the family is in a high state of anxiety. Even when the doctor solves the clinical problem, the family is likely to misunderstand much of the consultation. The conclusions family members draw from the expert opinion about other physicians, themselves, or the long-term care may be heard only by the counselor.

The chronic illness/acute doctor syndrome is one which is especially prevalent in medical centers where a great deal of training is done. Many of the seizure disorders, adjustment problems, affiliated learning dysfunctions, and family mismanagement can often be defined—transiently—but a long-term management plan is not specified, nor is the responsibility for its implementation clearly designated. Thus, the patient goes from doctor to doctor, accruing notes rather than planned interventions. Mental health planning needs to tie down relevant supports and interventions.

The misunderstanding/anger complex is one in which the physician does not clearly indicate his or her understanding and appreciation of the burden the family is carrying, however great or small it may actually be. Often when a family feels that the physician does not appreciate its struggles, its visits to the doctor turn into a series of demonstrations of the failure of the physician to adequately "treat" the illness, as well as various and sundry acts of noncompliance. This must be kept in mind when a lot of complaints are raised about medical care in the counseling situation.

The last complication is iatrogenic hopefulness. In other words, the support and hope that doctors have offered families about "things working out well" can, in some cases, mean that the family's tendency to define blame—within themselves, with doctors, or the child—is exacerbated whenever there is a change in seizure frequency or an unexpected complication.

A useful clinical attitude is optimistic fatalism. Denckla[39] applies this term to learning disabilities. It is useful, too, with epilepsy. An attitude of optimistic fatalism suggests, "You're stuck with this thing, and it may get better, and it may not"—but, optimistically, "Let's see how we can make the best of it."

This attitude helps make parents into clinical partners. They can collaborate in finding out the best way to manage the youngster's seizure disorder, either in regard to medication therapy, particular aspects of behavioral management, or schooling suggestions. Optimistic fatalism acknowledges a degree of uncertainty, but it is possible, over time, to discover the best guidelines for and strengths of a particular youngster.

Those cases with a poor prognosis need an alliance which accepts limitations. In poor prognosis cases, the clinical alliance and the family need to endure more clinical fluctuations, more poorly controlled periods of seizures, and more difficult behavioral and schooling questions that arise.

CONCLUSIONS

Work with a child with seizures must be based on a comprehensive diagnostic model. In addition to understanding the particular impact of the child's neurological problem and the youngster's cognitive and affective abilities, one must evaluate the impact of a chronic medical illness on a particular family system. Mental health professionals can best be prepared to treat the consequent problems by utilizing two conceptual models: (1) systems theory, and (2) problem definition and problem solving. Because of the long-term nature of the illness, it is often best to keep treatment plans to those that accomplish a clear goal in a relatively brief time. Additional interventions may then be coordinated with the family without creating another additional chronic and discouraging burden in the child's overall care.

REFERENCES

1. Livingston, S. The diagnosis of epilepsy, *Pediatric Annals*, 8:131-199, 1979.
2. Lombroso, C. T. *Convulsive Disorders in Newborns*. In: R. Thompson (ed.), *Pediatric Neurology and Neurosurgery*, New York: Spectrum Publications, 1978.
3. Whitehouse, D. Behavior and learning problems in epileptic children. *Behavioral Neuropsychiatry*, 7:23-29, 1970.
4. Harrison, R. M. and Taylor, D. Childhood seizures: A 25 Year Follow-up. *Lancet*, 1:948-951, 1976.
5. Ziegler, R. Psychological vulnerability in epilepsy. *Psychosomatics*, 20:145-148, 1979.
6. Kagan, J., Kearsley, R. and Zelazo, P. *Infancy*. Cambridge, MA: Harvard University Press, 1978.
7. Wender, P. H. Vicious and virtuous circles. *Psychiatry*, 31:314-324, 1968.
8. Hoffman, L., Deviation amplifying processes in natures groups. In: J. Haley (ed.), *Changing Families*, New York: Grune & Stratton, 1971.
9. Bateson, G. *Steps to an Ecology of Mind*. New York: Ballantine Books, 1972.
10. Asby, W. R. *Design for a Brain*, London: Science Paperbacks, 1965.
11. Geschwind, N. Borderland of neurology and psychiatry. In: D. Benson and D. Blumer (eds.), *Psychiatric Aspects of Neurological Disease*. New York: Grune & Stratton, 1975.
12. Whitehouse, op. cit.
13. Geist, R. Onset of chronic illness in children and adolescents. *Amer. Journal Orthopsychiatry*, 49:4-23, 1979.
14. Lezak, M. Living with the characterologically altered brain injured patient. *The Journal of Clinical Psychiatry*, 12:592-598, 1977.
15. Ward, F. and Bower, B. *A Study of Certain Social Aspects of Epilepsy in Childhood*. London: Spastics International Medical Publications, 1978.
16. Grunebaum, N. and Chassin, R. Relabeling and reframing reconsidered: The beneficial effects of a pathological label. *Family Process*, 17:449-456, 1978.
17. Tseng, W. S. and McDermott, J. Triaxial family classification, *J. of American Acad. of Child Psych.*, 18:22-43, 1979.
18. Jackson, D. D. and Yalom, I. Family interaction, family homeostasis, and some implications for conjoint family psychotherapy. In: J. H. Masserman (ed.), *Individual Family Dynamics*. New York: Grune & Stratton, 1959.

19. Minuchin, S., Rosman, R., and Baker, L. *Psychosomatic Families*. Cambridge: Harvard University Press, 1978.
20. Ackerman, N. *The Psychodynamics of Family Life*. New York: Basic Books, 1958.
21. Chess, S. The plasticity of human development. *J. of Amer. Acad. of Child Psychiatry*, 17:80-91, 1978.
22. Flavell, J. H. *The Developmental Psychology of Jean Piaget*. New York: Van Nostrand Reinhold Co., 1960.
23. Bruner, J. *Beyond the Information Given*. New York: W. W. Norton & Co., 1973.
24. Murphy, L. B. *Personality in Young Children*. New York: Basic Books, 1956.
25. Ziegler, R. Characterological adaptations to learning disorders. *J. of Learning Disabilities*. (in press).
26. Bandler, R. and Grinder, J. *The Structure of Magic (Vol. I)* Palo Alto: Science and Behavior Books, 1975.
27. Nicoli, A. Introduction. In: A. Nicoli (ed.), *The Harvard Guide to Modern Psychiatry*. Cambridge: The Belknap Press of Harvard University Press, 1978.
28. Rivines, T., Psychiatric effects of the anticonvulsant regimens. In: R. Shader (ed.), *Psychiatric Complications of Medical Drugs*. New York: Raven Press, 1979.
29. Koppitz, E. M. *The Bender Gestalt Test for Young Children*. New York: Grune and Stratton, 1963.
30. Reid, W. J. and Epstein, L. *Task Centered Casework*. New York: Columbia University Press, 1972.
31. Ziegler, R. Task focused therapy for children and parents, *Amer. J. Psychotherapy*, 34:107-118, 1980.
32. Mostofsky, D. and Balaschak, B. Psychobiological control of seizures. *Psychological Bulletin*, 4:723-750, 1977.
33. Shader, R. (ed.) *Manual of Psychiatric Therapeutics*. Boston: Little, Brown & Co., 1975.
34. Speck, R. V. and Rueveni, U. "Network therapy"—A developing concept. *Family Process*, 8:182-191, 1969.
35. Grass, E. Psychosocial impact on the patient and family unit. Part of a Symposium on the Awareness of Epilepsy, St. Joseph's Hospital and Medical Center, Phoenix, Arizona, Sept., 1978.
36. Voeller and Rothenberg, Psychosocial management of management in children. *Pediatrics*, 51:1072-81, 1973.
37. Ounsted, C. The hyperactive syndrome in epileptic children. *Lancet*, 2:303-311, 1955.
38. Winnicott, D. The theory of the parent-infant relationship. In: *The Maturational Processes and the Facilitating Environment*, New York: International Universities Press, Inc., 1965.
39. Denckla, M. Hyperactivity. Lecture at Children's Hospital Medical Center, Boston, January, 1979.

8

ADJUSTMENT TO DAILY LIVING

ROBERT T. FRASER, PH.D.
and
WAYNE R. SMITH, PH.D.

For the person with a seizure disorder, major life adjustment thrusts appear to be in the areas of vocational self-sufficiency, social adequacy, and the capacity for independent living. It is these areas that the epilepsy centers of Europe are emphasizing as they move toward deinstitutionalization of their former "colony" settings for people with epilepsy. Similarly, it is toward client adjustment in these areas that the health services professionals in the United States must direct their efforts.

"RELATED IMPAIRMENTS" AND LIFE ADJUSTMENT

As has been discussed in previous chapters of this book, it is not necessarily the seizures themselves but the various associated impairments that can present the greatest barriers to life adjustment for the person with epilepsy. Rodin, Shapiro, and Lennox[1] over five years (1970-74) classified patients seen at the Michigan Epilepsy Center (n = 369) into two major groups: those with epilepsy only and those with epilepsy and other associated handicaps (behavioral problems, intellectual disturbances or organic difficulties, other neurological handicaps); only 23 percent of this group were evaluated by Center staff as having epilepsy only.

The implications of such statistical comparison on a number of variables indicated that the "epilepsy only" group performs very similarly to members

The support of NIH Grant No. N 01-N5-6-2341, awarded by the National Institute of Neurological and Communicative Disorders and Stroke, PHS/DHEW, is acknowledged. Appreciation is also extended to Mrs. Helen M. Foutch for preparation of the manuscript and to the World Rehabilitation Fund, whose recent fellowship support is responsible for some of the information contained within the chapter.

of the general population, without any major difficulties in the work or educational settings. Conversely, it is those individuals with the associated difficulties, specifically neurological impairments and psychological problems, who encounter adjustment difficulties. It is this population that may promote any identifiable stigma attached to epilepsy by blaming seizures for the difficulties they encounter in life.[2] It is also for members of this group that the mental health professional will often be asked to provide services.

A comprehensive diagnostic foundation (see Chapter 6) is the first step in the planning of any intervention. The neurologist and neuropsychologist can aid in the formulation of an intervention by culling out the major difficulties affecting the individual with epilepsy. A neuropsychologist can be particularly helpful in providing discrimination between psychosocial and organic deficits relating to memory, problem solving, capacity for attention, and so on (see Chapter 5). The importance of diagnosis in vocational preparation will be discussed on pages 196-97.

VOCATIONAL PREPARATION

The job-related difficulties of the individual with epilepsy are well documented. A recent *Rehabilitation Brief*, for example, describes employer response to the job applicant with epilepsy:

> Few want to hire epileptics. In 1977, unemployment among epileptics was twice the national average and underemployment was even greater. In 1972, only 1.4 percent of all state vocational rehabilitation agency rehabilitants were epileptics. This had declined from 1.8 percent in 1950.[3]

More specifically, a review of employment studies on members of this population by the Epilepsy Foundation of America[4] indicates an unemployment rate for those in the labor force that varies between 20 and 25 percent. A recent study conducted in the State of Oregon,[5] based upon a sample of men aged 25 and over who were actively looking for work, revealed an unemployment rate of 19.5 percent; the authors indicate, however, that if those individuals with epilepsy who described themselves as "discouraged" or "disinterested" in a job search were included in the unemployment statistic, this rate would approximate 34 percent.

It is of special interest in this Oregon study that those groups having one or more grand mal or psychomotor seizures each year approximated a 50-percent unemployment rate. Having one of either type of seizure on a yearly basis appears to be the crucial factor in unemployment! This 50-percent unemployment rate halves for those groups having less than one grand mal or one psychomotor seizure each year. It is also of interest that within those groups having *more* than one psychomotor or grand mal seizure each year, the unemployment rate is not appreciably higher than 50 percent; there is not a linear correlation between seizure frequency and the unemployment rate.

Other employment-related problems exist in relation to underemployment and early withdrawal from the work force. Both the Oregon study,[6] and Rodin, Rennick, Dennerll, and Lin[7] have demonstrated that individuals with epilepsy tend to cluster toward the low skill ranges of the employment spectrum. Both the Oregon study and Farrago[8] also suggest early discouragement in relation to "job-getting" and withdrawal from active job search. Of course, this type of discouragement is a logical outcome of underemployment and long periods of unemployment

The National Epilepsy League[9] surveyed the needs of individuals with epilepsy by mailing a questionnaire to every fifteenth name on the roster of the League's pharmacy service. A total of 346 respondents (a response rate of 56 percent) identified vocational problems as some of the most important encountered by the person with epilepsy:

1. Discrimination in jobs was ranked as the most serious problem encountered by individuals with epilepsy (32 percent response rate);
2. Fifty percent indicated that epilepsy had created problems in procuring a job;
3. Job counseling was indicated as the service for which there was the greatest need (27 percent response rate), above the need for better medical care (22.5 percent)

In addition to the previously discussed unemployment data, the vocational problems as identified through this study provide further verification of this population's difficulties in the vocational area. Again, it should be emphasized that many from this group would have epilepsy and associated disabilities.

Issues in Vocational Adjustment

Basic issues that should be discussed in rehabilitation planning involving a person with epilepsy are seizure control, seizure frequency, and stress in relation to vocational activity. Questions relating to these areas are often presented by the individual with epilepsy, other members of the family, health service professionals, or employers.

Seizure Control. There has been a long-standing practice in the field of rehabilitation to wait for medical control of the seizures before undertaking any vocational intervention. This practice is often a real disservice to young adults with epilepsy. There is some evidence to indicate that persons with epilepsy often start considering the job market five to six years later than their peer group. For example, the mean age of vocational unit clients at the University of Washington Epilepsy Center was found to be 28 years, with approximately 40 percent having no prior work history.[10]

Since it is generally accepted that about 80 percent of those with epilepsy are competitively employable,[11] it behooves the rehabilitation counselor to get involved in vocational planning with the client as soon as possible. In cases where the client is too seizure-impaired for competitive employment, it may be possible to involve the individual in a prevocational work experience, or sheltered work program. A caution is that although a person is seizure-free at one point in time, there is no guarantee that the person will maintain this freedom from seizures at even a one-year follow-up.[12] Therefore, it is early involvement and a well-developed rehabilitation plan that will sustain the person with epilepsy to some degree of vocational stability.

Seizure Frequency. Depending on the type or pattern of the seizures, an individual can remain very employable despite frequent seizures (see pages 196-97). A more sophisticated neurological evaluation than the person has previously received may also result in dramatic seizure reduction through the effective use of a new anticonvulsant regimen. Finally, concentration on the work activity itself may have a therapeutic effect in reducing seizure activity. There are several studies conducted at Epi-Hab sites, sheltered industries which hire only people with epilepsy, that document the minimal amount of time lost due to seizures while on the job.[13,14] Seizures seem to occur more often during non-working hours or in periods following physical activity.[15]

Job-Related Stress. Another concern that tends to be overemphasized is the effect of stress on seizure activity. Although job-related stress can be a precipitant of seizures, this is not true for everyone with epilepsy. In many cases, it is more stressful for an individual to be jobless and confined to the home than to be involved in a work activity that could be construed as stressful. As an individual gets accustomed to a work setting and invested in the work activity, seizures initially exacerbated by the stress of a new work environment often gradually decrease. This phenomenon is often observed at our Center's work experience or job station sites.

The Importance of Vocational Counseling

As previously discussed, people with epilepsy form an underserved population in relation to vocational rehabilitation services. Reviews of percentage of rehabilitants by the national-state system of vocational rehabilitation indicate that greater percentages of clients with epilepsy were being rehabilitated during the 1960s than in the present decade.[16, 17] Scrutiny of intake statistics at our Center indicates that one of every two vocational clients had no prior contact with the state system of vocational rehabilitation.[18]

It appears that although vocational group counseling approaches have been successfully used with this population,[19, 20] follow-up data from the University of Washington Epilepsy Center indicated that clients tended to prefer individual vis-à-vis group vocational activities. Individual vocational counseling time consistently received above average Likert scale ratings (five-point rating scale), while group vocational activities only approximated average ratings. Given the multiplicity of problems affecting people with epilepsy, it seems quite logical that they will require sufficient "personal time" with a counselor to thoroughly explore not only their vocational plans but also critical psychosocial concerns. Two categories of counseling issues in which time is frequently invested by counselor and client include the areas of independence and acceptance of seizure status.

Independence. It can be very difficult for children and adults with epilepsy, as well as members of their families, to make an adjustment to this disability. The individual with epilepsy can physically appear, and often perform, like anybody else, except during that period of time in which a seizure occurs. The fact that the seizures do occur, however, often results in parents or significant others expecting less of the person in relation to home chores, school achievement, involvement in social and recreational activities, and so on. In many cases, a person's decision-making capabilities are preempted by members of the family. In these situations, much of the counseling relationship involves inviting the client, with the family's support, to begin more independent decision-making. In a supportive and optimistic fashion, the counselor assists the client in vocational goal-planning. Other avenues that lead toward client independence include work experience programs that provide a reality base to vocational exploration, and various programs, such as social skills training, which reduce the client's social isolation and augment the value of the counseling relationship.

Acceptance. Acceptance of seizure status does not mean "resignation" to a lifetime of seizures, but rather acceptance of the fact that while the individual is subject to seizures, "working with and around" them is an effective method of coping compared to denial, which is a pathological defense and prevents dealing with reality. It should be emphasized that acceptance of seizure status does not necessarily mean disclosure of seizure status to the employer. Disclosure of seizure status is a very individual choice, and for some individuals (who have their seizures only at night or very infrequently) it can be very appropriate to not discuss the disability with an employer (see page 197). Persons can be encountered, however, who, despite frequent and severe seizure activity, persist in not discussing the situation with employers, refuse to admit that they shouldn't drive, or would rather be accused of abusing drugs than have an employer know that they are experiencing seizures.

If individuals are accepting of their current seizure status, the person with whom they are interacting tends to be more at ease in relation to the condition. When a person can comfortably and succinctly discuss epilepsy with an employment interviewer, the interviewer becomes more assured that medical status will be understandable to the line supervisor. If counselor and client can successfully work towards the client's acceptance of the disability, the client is better prepared to modify the uncertainties and negative attitudes that are encountered in the social, educational, and vocational arenas.

Vocational Evaluation Concerns

In assisting the client to identify vocational goals, most of the standardized psychological tests are applicable for use with clients with epilepsy. There are, however, a number of clinical cautions which should be offered to the counselor. In the area of interest inventories, for example, many young adults will have difficulties responding to items because of their lack of life exposure as compared to groups on which tests were standardized. An allowance must be made for possible test score differential, and tests must be interpreted from this reference point. If a client is not interested or capable of college work (interests routinely assessed by the Strong-Campbell,[21] Kuder DD,[22] etc.), the use of a checklist inventory which directly lists a large number of specific work activities (for example, the Gordon Occupational Check List[23]) can be more appropriate. A pictorial interest inventory (for example, the Reading Free Vocational Interest Inventory[24]) can be used when educational deficiencies and intellectual/neurological impairments make use of the others impossible.

Assessing aptitude and achievement capabilities with people who have epilepsy is often quite difficult. Efforts made to establish some standardized index of academic achievement or potential can be meaningless. The problem is that young persons with epilepsy may be unfairly assigned to special education classes, may miss large amounts of school time due to seizures, or may have had a number of problems in school due to the effects of subclinical absence seizures not apparent to the teacher but interfering with the learning process.[25] Although scoring poorly on a standardized achievement test, a number of clients with epilepsy will perform adequately or on an above-average level following remedial work at a community college or adult education program.

In administering aptitude tests to persons with epilepsy, it should be realized that low-level familial expectancies, lack of test and work experience, fear of triggering a seizure through exertion, and neurological impairments (for example, poor attention span) can adversely affect performance on timed aptitude tests. On tasks involving motor speed and coordination, the client with epilepsy is often at a special disadvantage due to the effects of seizures and anticonvulsants over time, not to mention a prevalent lack of involvement in sports activities in which motor skills are refined. In administering motor aptitude tests, the Institute for Epilepsy in Heemstede, Holland, uses not only a series of trials but also a pacing system (via individual headset) to enable a person to achieve a more "competitive, yet personally tolerable" level of performance. In aptitude assessment at our Center, a motor aptitude test is also administered several times with intermittent reinforcement and pacing in order that a more accurate evaluation of performance capabilities can be made.

In assisting a person with epilepsy to identify specific aptitudes and interest, "in vivo" work experience programs are often the best method of concomitantly assessing capabilities while exploring different types of work interests. Different types of work experience programs will be discussed in detail on pages 199-200.

Working with the Neuropsychologist

The report of a neuropsychologist can be invaluable for vocational planning with the client who has epilepsy. In a population that is afflicted with sundry disabilities in addition to the epilepsy—intellectual deficits, various forms of brain impairment, and psychosocial difficulties—it becomes extremely important to have objective data that accurately assess the psychological and social functions of the client in order to know which problems to confront and which to work around.

In addition to the general standardized measures, such as the Wechsler Adult Intelligence Scale, the Minnesota Multiphasic Personality Inventory, and the Lateral Dominance Examination,[26] the specialized neuropsychological measures developed by Drs. Halstead and Reitan usually form the core of the neuropsychological battery. These measures are used to discriminate between normal performance and that of brain-impaired populations. More recently, Dodrill[27] has identified a battery of 16 discriminative measures which are useful in differentiating the neuropsychological performance of those with epilepsy from that of the normal populace. In vocational counseling with persons with epilepsy, it can be very important to understand the cumulative effects of seizures and anticonvulsants on brain functions such as attention to task, reaction time, and perceptual and motor functions. A simple determination of "brain damage" (if this is the case) is not enough. The counselor involved in vocational planning must have more specific information regarding both residual adaptive skills and deficiency areas. The battery recently established by Dodrill provides a standardized group of measures to be used in evaluating persons with epilepsy, taking into account those factors that unequally influence psychological and social performance of persons with a history of this disorder.

The Importance of Seizure-related Information in Vocational Counseling

A major variable involved in vocationally working with people having epilepsy is the ability of the counselor to gather complete seizure-related information. The most obvious data to be gathered is the seizure type and frequency with an accurate description of the seizure activity itself. This information is often impossible to secure from the client and must therefore be secured from a family member, neurologist, or significant other. There is a substantial proportion of people with epilepsy who have no idea of "how they look" during a seizure. A seizure occurrence can be dramatically magnified in their minds. Understanding of what does happen during the seizure not only dispels fantasy and tends to improve the client's self-presentation, but can be vital information for the employer—for example, does the person fall to the ground, lose consciousness, maintain physical control, etc.?

Other important information relates to precipitants of seizures. Are there particular factors which seem to trigger seizure activity in the client? For some with epilepsy, precipitants of seizure activity can include fatigue, anxiety, fevers, alcohol intake, or flickering lights. It should be emphasized, however, that every case is individual and many people with epilepsy have no identifiable seizure precipitants. Other pre-ictal seizure information concerns whether the individual has a dependable warning on the day of the seizure (nausea, for example) or has a consistent aura (the aura is the early part of the seizure, in which the person is conscious and may be experiencing tingling or other unusual sensations—see page 11). For some individuals, a dependable warning on the day of a seizure may make it judicious to take a sick day. A dependable seizure aura may provide time to assume a "safe" position (sitting or lying down), thus minimizing injury possibilities in the work setting.

Information that is often overlooked in the vocational interview concerns the existence of the individual's specific seizure pattern. It is obvious that if a person's seizures, even though relatively frequent, occur in a pattern that does not involve normal work hours, the person generally would be considered more employable. Similarly, if a person has several seizures a month with the seizures clustering over a period of hours or a day, employment prospects might also be improved. The context in which seizures occur (for example, certain stressful situations) must also be explored, as this is often the basis for a counseling intervention. One could try to arrange job hours so as to avoid seizure patterns.

Finally, the consequences of an individual having a seizure must be examined. The amount of recovery time that is necessary prior to return to work can be a key factor not only in securing a job, but also in maintaining the position. After a severe seizure, some individuals can return to work in an hour, while many others cannot return until the next day. An individual's reaction to a seizure incident varies considerably (embarrassment, withdrawal, anger, denial, for example) and should be addressed in the course of rehabilitation planning and counseling. If the person has chosen to disclose seizure status to an employer (see pages 201-202), it can help the applicant's case if it can be established that there is no history of work-related injuries or accidents.

Vocational Group Approaches

There are several vocational group approaches that are used routinely in the rehabilitation field and in job preparation of the hard-core unemployed which also have applicability in the field of epilepsy rehabilitation. Vocational group activity can be very helpful in readying the person with epilepsy for the employment market and providing support in the job search. Following is a synopsis of some vocational group approaches.

Vocational Exploration Group. A vocational exploration group[28, 29] involves a small group approach and a structured interaction between peer group members that aids them in clarifying job or educational goals. Much of the group activity involves work-related values clarification, and materials are provided which assist in this process. Research completed with "hard-core unemployed" indicates that group members obtained twice the number of jobs as did controls and also had significantly higher employability perceptions. Vocational naiveté is a common problem among young adults with epilepsy. The vocational exploration group structure can assist such individuals toward developing and refining job goals in a basically supportive group environment.

Job-Seeking Skills Programs. Given the social deficits, lack of work experience, and the associated disabilities experienced by many young adults with epilepsy, involvement in a job-seeking skills program often becomes imperative. Most of the existing job-seeking skill programs parallel or are modifications of the program developed by the Minnesota Rehabilitation Center.[30] The skills that are taught or coached can include application completion, telephone "cold calling" of employers, résumé development, identification of leads, and employment interviewing (videotaped). Discussion of seizure status and completion of the application are areas in which many young adults with epilepsy can require extensive coaching (see pages 201-202). Job-seeking skill programs can involve one day to three weeks, but a succinct program can be effective in a one-and-a-half day period for a group of eight to ten clients. Many of those with epilepsy will require repeated coaching due to additional disabilities (for example, brain impairment).

Job-Finding Club. The job-finding club group format was originally described by Azrin, Flores, and Kaplan[31] and has been widely and successfully used with both rehabilitation and hard-core unemployed persons. At our Center, job club consists of weekly two-hour meetings for a group of eight to 12 job-ready clients. The first part of the meeting consists of sharing job leads and group "brainstorming" of job ideas for each participant. Other job search concerns (transportation and health insurance, for example) are discussed quite often. In the second section of the meeting, different community employers are involved in explaining access routes into their respective companies and job applicant characteristics that each company finds desirable. This type of group setting builds a family-type support structure, provides an arena for problem-solving, and involves aspects of implicit and explicit confrontation in regard to each person's job search, thus building confidence. The presence of the employer and the sharing of job leads reinforce attendance at the job club meetings. Many of these employers hire job club members or later become employment contacts for group members. The group leader establishes the expectancy for a certain number of weekly employer contacts by each participant.

Other job club formats involve daily group meetings with a specified number of activities (for example, daily phone calls made to employers). It becomes obvious that the more group support provided and the more frequent the contact with potential employers, the greater is the probability of securing employment.

The Role of the Family in Vocational Rehabilitation

In working toward successful vocational rehabilitation of the young adult with epilepsy, it is often important to involve the family. In a recent study at our center[32] parents endorsed the following two problem areas most frequently on a family problems rating form:

1. Not knowing how to effectively encourage son or daughter to be as independent as possible.
2. Son or daughter is having difficulty finding or keeping a job.

Although parents recognize "independence" and "job-finding" as desirable goals for their offspring, they often impede efforts in these areas through their fears and anxieties about the well-being of the young adult. This is, of course, understandable; however, the young adult must engage in personal "job-getting" or "self-establishment" efforts if any progress is to be made in these areas. Having shown their children how to take the reasonable precautions, parents must be counseled to help their son or daughter become involved in some "risk-taking" activities (for example, taking the bus alone) despite lack of full control of seizures. Parent counseling sessions, in addition to dealing with the overprotection issue, can emphasize parental acceptance of a son's or daughter's seizure status, establishing realistic expectations within the family context and encouraging regularity in relation to diet and rest.

In relation to job search assistance, simply freeing the phone for certain periods during the work week to allow their son or daughter to contact employers or receive calls can be very helpful. This type of support, coupled with frequent verbal encouragement, considerably facilitates job search success.

Maximizing Vocational Potential: A Placement Continuum

For the person with epilepsy who is just entering the labor force or reentering after a number of years, there are several steps that can be taken to enable adjustment to a particular job or to work in general. Following are some steps in the placement process.

Work Sample or Work Experience. In this step, the person works at either simulation of real work activity (work sample), or actually engages in one or more types of real work activity in a sheltered workshop or as a volunteer (in a hospital setting, university setting, or nonprofit agency). Volunteer status can guarantee insurance coverage. This type of program can provide an individual the opportunity to assess both capabilities and interests in relation to various types of work activity.

Job Tryout. In the job tryout, a person is evaluated on a job in the competitive market. This might involve one day or several weeks and is often subsidized by a rehabilitation agency. If a client's wages are paid by a rehabilitation agency during this period, difficulties with unions, insurance coverage, and other company objections can often be circumvented. Commonly, there is a "good faith" agreement between rehabilitation agency and a firm to hire a person if the tryout appears satisfactory (tryouts may be abused in favor of the company and must be carefully monitored by counselor or placement specialist). There is a psychological advantage to this type of placement approach; it becomes difficult for the employing firm to reject a person who has been on a job tryout for several weeks. The federal government has a "selective certification" program that is akin to a job tryout inasmuch as formal testing requirements are waived for a person with a disability and the person is provided 700 hours to establish competence on the job. At our Center this system has been an excellent vehicle for enabling young adults with epilepsy to gain access to the federal civil service system.

On-the-job Training. This type of training is a negotiated program between an employer and the rehabilitation or manpower agency (for example, Comprehensive Employment and Training Act Agency) in which the trainee's salary is shared by both parties. At the end of the customary three-to-six-month training period, the employer is committed (although not legally) to retain the employee and assume sole responsibility for wages. This type of training program is an excellent option for those rehabilitation clients who learn by doing and require more immediate financial reinforcement. On-the-job training programs provide the counselor with a negotiating basis for job development contact with employers. Counselors should also monitor this type of program to be certain that the trainee is learning a specific set of skills and thus ensure his or her continued employability.

Approaching the Employer

Although there is some evidence that employer attitudes toward hiring an individual with epilepsy are changing positively,[33] a number of studies also exist suggesting that changing these hiring attitudes can be quite difficult.[34, 35, 36] Perhaps the most accurate assessment of the situation was made by Zielinski, who stated, "Although employers may express quite positive opinions about epileptics, they are often afraid to hire persons known to them as having even rare epileptic seizures."[37] It would seem that if the person with epilepsy is to successfully procure work, the manner in which the employer is approached is very important.

In some cases, the rehabilitation agency will make an initial job development contact with an employer. The San Antonio Training and Placement Services (TAPS) unit for people with epilepsy limits their initial employer contact to 20 minutes and expands the presentation to 35 minutes if the employer seems particularly interested.[38] Although a rehabilitation agency may be interested in developing a specific job for a client, this can be done within the context of a broader program presentation. The agency should first investigate employer needs (manpower and other) and then emphasize the services that it can provide (Affirmative Action Assistance, transportation problem-solving, pre-screened applicants, or on-the-job training, for example). It should be emphasized that "reasonable accommodation" and accessibility issues are minimal for members of this populace.

Dealing with Employer Objections. It is usually not advisable to introduce potential employer objections into the job development conversation, but nevertheless the agency representative should be prepared to deal with these issues as they arise. In general, studies indicate that the job performance of the employee with epilepsy is equal to or better than the non-disabled employee in areas such as productivity,[39] and other studies document the minimal amount of time lost due to seizures on the job.[40, 41] In relation to accidents on the job, Sands,[42] in reviewing workers' compensation claims in the state of New York, indicates that sneezing and coughing appear to cause twice the number of compensable accidents as those attributable to seizures.

Other employer concerns involve Workers' Compensation or fear that the employee with epilepsy will have a seizure-related accident causing permanent disability. Hiring a person with epilepsy does not, of itself, cause rate hikes, as these rates are simply based upon the employing company's industrial classification or overall accident experience. Health insurance costs are usually linked to age and sex characteristics in larger companies, while among smaller companies (less than 100 employees) health expense claim experiences are generally pooled. Again, no company is penalized by health insurance rate increases in hiring a person with a disability. In approximately 21 states, Workers' Compensation Second Injury Funds appear to restrict the liability of the employer to the amount of accident compensation that would be equitable if the preexisting seizure condition had not been present—that is, *not* to the compound effect of the injury and the preexisting condition.

For a more complete discussion of Workers' Compensation, see the resource manual *New Directions in Epilepsy*,[43] and for more information on handling employer objections read the work of Sinick.[44]

Disclosure of Seizure Status. In approaching the work world, disclosure of seizure status is a very individual concern and strategies will vary. For some individuals with complete seizure control, nocturnal seizures, or seizures that will not occur at work, it may not be necessary to tell an employer.

In other cases, the frequency or severity of seizures is such that it would not be in the interest of the person with epilepsy not to discuss the condition with an employer. According to a study by Perlman,[45] 68 percent of those with epilepsy prefer that their employer understand their condition.

At our Center, we generally advise our clients not to write down "epilepsy" on the application form but to wait for the interview if they wish to discuss the disability. In the interview session, after job-related skills and abilities have been described, individuals are coached to describe their seizures clearly and succinctly in terms the employer will understand. Terms like "grand mal," "petit mal," "spells," and other foreign or confusing terms are to be avoided—what actually occurs during the seizure is the key! The person who can discuss a seizure condition with self-assurance does much to assuage employer concerns.

Some workers in the field advise having the client's doctor contact the prospective employer to discuss the job and the client from the standpoint of safety, performance, and absenteeism. This should be done only with the client's agreement and by a doctor having a clear understanding of the job environment and work demands.

Acclimation to the Job

The first few months on a job can be a difficult period of time for the employee with epilepsy. It can be especially helpful if a supervisor or trusted co-worker understands the specifics of a person's seizure condition and what to do if a seizure occurs. A rehabilitation or other counselor who is knowledgeable about epilepsy can often help by giving a short educational presentation about epilepsy to a group of co-workers or members of a department. People who are able to accept their own seizure conditions may still have difficulty dealing with the reactions of co-workers. Short-term counseling directed at dealing with job-related concerns can be helpful. Excessive discussion of one's seizure condition on the job site is to be avoided. Epilepsy and related problems should be discussed with a rehabilitation or other trusted counselor. Another approach to handling problems on the job could be weekly peer group sessions as a post-employment rehabilitation service.

Post-placement Services

Follow-up is generally considered an important service in the field of vocational rehabilitation. The problems associated with epilepsy, however, render follow-up a critical client service. At our Center, follow-up received some of the highest client ratings as contrasted with various other vocational services.[46] Although about 70 percent of our clients have seizures on a monthly basis and 95 percent on a yearly basis, less than five individuals over a four-year period have lost jobs due to seizure-related incidents, and even in these few cases seizures were not always the sole reason for dismissal. Our major concern in relation to client job retention is interpersonal or emotional difficulties on the job. A substantial amount of time has been invested by our counseling staff in individual follow-up counseling sessions and job site interventions. Efforts to sustain a job maintenance or career enrichment group have not met with success; the national TAPS program seems to have had similar difficulties maintaining these kinds of groups. After involvement in a day's work, a job-related group situation seems to have little appeal.

More recently, efforts to establish social or recreational "after-hours" groups seem to be meeting with more interest, while still being supportive of a job adjustment thrust. Sands and Radin[47] report success in establishing peer group support systems for employed ex-mentally ill rehabilitants.

Involvement in this type of group reduces social isolation, abets interpersonal functioning, and can be viewed as a more "normal" activity for a working person. Problem-solving and job adjustment difficulties can still be broached in a more informal manner in these social settings with either peers or participating professional staff.

SOCIAL SKILLS

As more is learned about the natural course of seizure disorders and the process of their rehabilitation, evidence is mounting that the individual's adjustment to the disorder is often less dependent on the number and severity of the seizures than on a variety of attitudinal and psychosocial factors: fear of public censure, loss of self-esteem, social isolation, the belief that it is impossible to lead a normal life, and intrusive feelings of frustration, hopelessness, and despair. As previously discussed, these psychosocial factors appear to show a greater association to vocational adjustment than does seizure frequency.[48, 49, 50]

Several reports document seizure disorder patients' poor social tension management and problem-solving skills, as well as a high incidence of passivity and depression.[51, 52] These psychosocial deficits are particularly apparent in patients with long-standing uncontrolled seizures,[53, 54, 55, 56] although there is significant variability among different seizure types.[57]

The skills training or psychoeducational approach[58, 59] to treating these psychosocial problems rests on a central tenet of behavior therapy—namely, that all our behavior, including thoughts and feelings, is learned, and generally unintentionally learned (unlike the popular view of learning as a purely

204 EPILEPSY: A HANDBOOK FOR THE MENTAL HEALTH PROFESSIONAL

intentional process). For the most part, this learning has developed over a period of years through a series of transactions with important people in our lives. Dysphoric moods, self-defeating thoughts, and social distress are therefore learned responses and can be replaced by learning more adaptive responses. Patients can learn more effective mood management skills (giving oneself periodic rewards, anticipating the effects of setbacks, and reducing life pressures) by learning to replace self-defeating thoughts with productive and rewarding thoughts and developing the social skills necessary to feel confident and valued in social situations.[60, 61, 62] Reports of this type of approach taken in individual therapy suggest promising results for chronic seizure disorder patients, [63, 64, 65, 66] but this section will focus on group-taught skills teaching.

Rationale for Skills Training Groups

It should be noted that we are referring in this section to *chronic* seizure disorder patients—those who have had to deal with the intrusive effects of having seizures for approximately six months or longer. As with a wide variety of chronic illnesses, this is often how long it takes to develop a stable and enduring pattern of behaviors in anticipation of and in response to having seizures. A large majority of the seizure-disorder patients now being treated by the comprehensive epilepsy programs and private neurologists are those who have had seizures since birth or adolescence. It is within this group that a failure to learn adaptive social and self-management skills, which results in the most apparent psychosocial problems, is clearest. Factors most likely related to this failure to learn include the absence of appropriate models for effectively handling seizure consequences, and long-term isolation from the multitude of casual social situations in which skillful social discourse and transaction are learned.

In addition, these patients carry with them a learning history characterized by the environment's responses to their "out-of-control" or disinhibited seizure behavior. This history often results in a rich repertoire of avoidance behaviors that are initially elicited unwillingly by parental concerns for their child's well-being and inadvertently maintained by physician's prescriptions to "avoid stress." The development of such avoidance behaviors is further reinforced by peers who attribute their friend's unexplainable seizure behavior to global traits such as "craziness," "attention-seeking," or "helplessness."

Because of the nature of the disorder itself, patients often naturally develop the perception of themselves as powerless to control important aspects of what is commonly referred to as "voluntary" behavior. Repeated exposure to noxious events viewed as outside of voluntary control can lead to feelings of hopelessness and avoidance of prudent risk-taking. Consequently, proficient adaptive skills are never learned.[67] The skills required to effectively manage the environment's responses to a person's "out of control" behavior are even less likely to develop in this context. It is the learned avoidance responses and failure to gain access to situations for learning adaptive social tension management and problem-solving skills that we encounter as the factors most directly related to the psychosocial dysfunction of chronic seizure disorder patients.

In this context, the applicability of skills training procedures for chronic seizure disorder patients is perhaps more understandable. If sense of self-control is impaired, individuals can be taught to maximize the control that they do have through the teaching and training, for example, of approaches to anticipating troublesome situations and new routines for engaging in productive problem solving. Through practice and discussion, patients can learn to become more skillful at clarifying and appropriately articulating their wishes. The process of enhancing a person's skill is the logical solution to his or her impaired self-esteem and feelings of helplessness and hopelessness.

The additional benefits of working with chronic seizure disorder patients in groups (see Chapter 6) have been noted in other less structured therapy groups;[68, 69, 70, 71] most notably, the fact that groups foster a sense of community and develop a life reference point. Different members of the group can be used to generate and model appropriate responses to seizure-related situations.

Structure of Skills Training Classes

Some comments on the general structure of skills training classes may be useful before we describe some of the specific classes developed by a group of psychologists and social workers at our Center. First, there are a few principles about fostering behavior change and skill acquisition that have come out of the skills training literature: The behavioral goals of any skills training class should ideally be clearly articulated, specific, and tailored as far as possible to each participant's situation—but, above all, attainable. There needs to be a certain amount of individual assessment through, for example, checklists of problematic situations, diary-keeping, or role-playing. Likelihood of skill acquisition is increased to the extent that each patient knows what skills he or she needs to acquire; this means a balance between making the goals general enough to incorporate the needs of all the patients in the class and yet tailoring the goals specifically to each patient.

The other element crucial to success is practice—through role-playing in class, structured homework assignments, and individual behavior change projects. There is evidence, for example, that understanding the principles of assertive behavior, mood management, or relaxation is not as strongly related to skill acquisition and behavior change as is performing the behaviors through role-plays, "in vivo" or in imagination.[72, 73]

Our Center has experimented with a number of skills training classes based on the above principles, typically employing eight weekly meetings of one-and-a-half hours each for its adult outpatients. Groups were limited to patients with no more than moderate cognitive deficits or impulse control problems.

Relevant Skills Training Classes

In this section, specific skills training classes that appear relevant to persons with epilepsy will be discussed.

Relaxation Training Class. The fact that many seizures are believed to be stress-related suggests the relevance of a relaxation training class, which teaches standard relaxation, desensitization, and cognitive self-control techniques (see Chapters 2 and 6) in order to foster effective tension control.[74] In addition, sensitizing the patient to the varying degrees of stress in commonly encountered situations may be helpful; this could be accomplished by keeping a diary and rating levels of experienced distress. A word of caution is necessary, however, with regard to using some relaxation techniques in a group format for chronic seizure disorder patients. There is some evidence to suggest that relaxation techniques which do not maintain a mental focus for the patient can lower seizure threshold.[75]

Assertiveness Class. Many persons who are not burdened by chronic illness frequently avoid expressing their wishes or making requests of others. People with epilepsy seem to have particular difficulty in asking for assistance, especially when it necessitates disclosure of their seizure condition. A class in assertiveness, descriptions of which are scattered through the research literature,[76, 77, 78] can easily be adapted for the special, as well as the more routine, problems chronic seizure disorder patients encounter.

Conversation Skills Class. A conversation skills class which allows patients to pinpoint deficient interpersonal skills can be invaluable for members of a populace that has been developmentally sheltered and, in adulthood, often socially isolated. Areas covered in this class can include introducing new topics, ending conversations, or asking questions and paraphrasing. Ample opportunity is also provided to practice these skills not only in role-playing situations, but in specific homework assignments (say good morning to the bus driver; call directory assistance to ask for several area codes). Role-playing and homework combine to gradually increase conversation skills and desensitize patients to the interpersonal risks involved in forming new friendships.

Mood Management Class. Many people become sad and listless at times for no apparent reason, but individuals show a wide variety of responses to this experience. Some respond only with increased feelings of frustration, self-denigration, and helplessness, while others seem to have their own routines for pulling themselves out of their depressed mood before it develops into a full-scale clinical depression. These routines may include "giving oneself a break" from time pressures, engaging in or planning some highly pleasant event, changing the reiterating thoughts from depression-engendering thoughts ("I'm getting less and less done") to competence-engendering thoughts ("What I am accomplishing now is really good work"). Chronic seizure disorder patients frequently show deficits in such mood management routines, likely due to their learning over long periods of time that they have relatively little control over important aspects of their voluntary behavior. A mood management class might teach various techniques such as scheduling pleasant events,[79] or thought stoppage,[80] in order to encourage more skillful control over dysfunctional moods.

Memory-Training Class. Perhaps the skills training class which has been most enthusiastically endorsed by our Center's patients, and yet the effects of which are the most difficult to document, is a memory training class which teaches habits that foster systematic approaches to acquiring and retrieving information. The memory deficits of persons with epilepsy,[81] as well as the difficulties inherent in teaching classes on memory techniques,[82] are well documented.

Class sessions can be organized around three basic steps in remembering:

1. Securing the initial information;
2. Linking the information with other familiar concepts and using mnemonic devices;
3. Retrieving the information when necessary.

Special emphasis is placed on covert verbal repetition, series of self-directed questions and answers to focus attention on important aspects of the task at hand, the routine use of calendars, efficient note-taking, and planning and scheduling daily activities. Homework assignments may include planning daily activities for a week, recording incidents of forgetting, taking notes on the evening T.V. news, or meeting strangers and remembering their names (telephone operators, salesclerks) without writing them down. A crucial aspect of training individuals to use these memory aids is to teach patients to recognize the discriminative cues indicating when to employ a particular strategy. It is the basic difficulty of "remembering how to remember" that makes training and homework so important in this class.

Problem-Solving Skills. One of the most promising skills training classes appears to be a class which teaches problem-solving skills. As with memory deficits, problem-solving deficits are sometimes only minimally responsive to skills teaching remediation due to the underlying brain dysfunction. In our experience, however, it appears that many patients initially do not know how to remember, nor do they know how to problem solve, but with persistent training these same patients can learn not only when, but also how, to solve their personal problems. Problem solving abilities usually refer to abstract reasoning and the ability to make judgments in complex, novel situations—abilities which are frequently compromised by mild to moderate cerebral dysfunction.[83] Personal problem-solving requires a variety of additional skills. These include:

1. The ability to inhibit the immediate responses to the problem (even though the individual is experiencing distress);
2. Analytic abilities of judging behavior-consequence relationships and abstracting the relevant features from an ongoing set of events;
3. The ability to reflect upon, reify, and categorize one's own behavior in terms of discrete responses to the problem situation.

D'Zurilla and Goldfried[84] have reviewed the findings regarding problem-solving skills, and Goldfried and Davison[85] provide lucid, step-by-step descriptions of a problem-solving procedure that has been employed in a skills training class for chronic seizure patients.[86, 87] Patients first learn to problem solve with hypothetical, but commonly experienced problems (for example, whether or not to move out of their parents' house, or how to handle a patronizing colleague at work). Later, the patient's own problems are used to practice the problem-solving skills in the group, with gradually less prompting by the teacher. The result, after many sessions, is a highly structured, action-oriented group therapy.

Management of Leisure Time. As young adults move into residences of their own and begin new jobs, judicious use of leisure time can help them combat loneliness and keep their social needs from intruding into the work setting. Areas to be covered in a leisure-time class can include vacation planning; identifying abilities that can be developed for various activities, games, and hobbies suited to certain interests; the city or community as an entertainment resource; or dining out and the social etiquette involved.

Human Relationships and Sexuality. This class subsumes subject matter such as developing a relationship, expectations and change in the relationship, privacy in the relationship, physical and emotional components of sexuality, and awareness of sexual aids or devices. At the Epilepsy Day Care Center in Hvidovre, Denmark, clients are subject to an interview at intake and assigned to one of two groups, a basic sex education or a more advanced relationships discussion group, based upon cognitive level and prior sexual experience.[88] This type of structuring seems to have enabled members of both groups to derive more from a program in this area.

Further Applications and Conclusions

The above is not, of course, an exhaustive list of all potential skills training classes appropriate for chronic seizure disorder patients—the basic format could be extended to a number of additional areas. For instance, accurate information regarding the number of seizures which occur between clinic visits is a major problem for physicians, who need this information to accurately adjust anticonvulsant medications. It is possible that some of the methods for training individuals how to monitor and record their behavior may be applied with significant benefit to adult seizure disorder patients.[89]

Another area for application of the skills training approach involves adapting the parent training literature to teaching parents how they may influence their sons and daughters to become more self-sufficient. Failure to gain independence on the part of the young adult seizure-disorder patient is often blamed on an overly protective parent, but this too can be viewed as parents' failure to learn a special set of skills. These skills involve the ability of a parent to protect but still support and encourage independent activity on the part of a son or daughter. These skills can be taught, as preliminary reports suggest,[90] with some degree of success.

Social skills training classes hold significant promise in working with people with epilepsy. In order to be effective, a skills training procedure, as in any form of therapy or counseling, must exert a significant influence over relevant aspects of the patient's life. The group skills training approach, particularly on a once-a-week outpatient basis, requires consistent, active involvement on the part of the patient. Involvement in social skills training cannot be viewed as a quick therapeutic panacea.

There is no question that substantial progress has been made in the social skills area. In a number of instances, however, social skills therapists will still have to rely on their best judgment until more thorough research and evaluation are available on the effectiveness of various new strategies.

INDEPENDENT LIVING SKILLS

Independent living means living outside an institution and within the community. Although the concept of independent living for those with disabilities has existed for some time, it is only within the last several years that the behavioral emphasis on teaching a wide spectrum of discrete independent living skills has become more formalized. An indication of the interest in this area is the success of the 1977 White House Conference on Independent Living for Handicapped Individuals. While definitions of independent living tend to vary, the underlying tenet involves the "ability of the severely disabled person to participate actively in society: to work, to own a home, to raise a family, etc."[91] From a vocational rehabilitation perspective, although independent living skills are not "mainstream" vocational, Krantz[92] emphasizes that these skills must be possessed by a person at some minimal level of competency in order that employment be sustained. Although overlap can exist between social skills and independent living skills, independent living skills tend to involve a very basic level of functioning in the community as contrasted with the previously discussed social skills.

Rationale

Much of the rationale for making independent living skills training available for people with epilepsy, especially young adults, parallels the reasons for teaching social skills. Basically, it is an effort to overturn the "learned helplessness" that is frequently observed in the young adult with a chronic seizure disorder. In Sutton, Smith, and Fraser's study,[93] parents cited their inability to encourage independence in their offspring with seizures as the most significant problem in their family. Many parents, in attempting to deal with this cyclic, sporadically disabling, condition of epilepsy, have difficulty establishing reasonable expectations for a son or daughter either inside or outside the home. Other evidence suggests that dependence in offspring with epilepsy may not be a function of the parents, but nevertheless the excessive dependency of the young upon their parents was affirmed.[94]

At our Center the mean age of the clients seen by the vocational unit is 28. Many of these clients have never left home and lack a number of independent living skills. It becomes quite obvious that if these individuals are to succeed vocationally, independent living skills training in areas such as use of public transportation, financial budgeting, and securing an apartment become crucial. For other individuals with severe seizure disorders, the issue is not necessarily work, but simply achieving a greater degree of self-esteem and life satisfaction; independent living skills help achieve these goals.

Structure of Independent Living Skills Training

Much of the structure for the training of independent living skills parallels that described for social skills training: clearly articulated and attainable goals, an individual assessment at intake, and the crucial element of practice. Independent living skills are taught in a variety of settings such as day-care centers for people with epilepsy,[95] within the local epilepsy association,[96] or within the person's home by independent living specialists or home health care teachers. It can often be more effective to teach independent living skills in smaller groups than are used in the social skills program, with as few as two or three students per group. This seems to facilitate the learning process when the class involves some more complex material and various equipment (as in a cooking class) or the class lesson is being given within the local community (as in a shopping trip). Other independent living classes, such as grooming, can normally be taught to a larger group of eight to 12, in the same format as the social skills training.

Relevant Independent Living Skills Classes

There are a number of independent living skill courses that are very relevant to people with epilepsy. Given the social isolation and dependency that can be encountered with this group, some basic courses on aspects of grooming and upkeep of physical appearance can be important. Another basic but valuable course can involve clothing (styles, selection, care, budget resources) and laundering. As young adults begin jobs and move toward independent living, a very immediate concern becomes that of moving out of their parents' home. A course that can be very helpful for these individuals involves living alternatives (shared housing, rooming houses, and so on) and aspects of the apartment search (an overview of neighborhoods, "where to look," itemized costs). An instructional unit that complements the course on living residences involves home equipment (necessary utensils or appliances, purchasing, safety features, types of controls) and obtaining furniture (friends and family as a resource, necessary furnishings, sources of inexpensive furniture). Another skills unit that relates to the home involves housekeeping and home maintenance (acceptable levels of home cleanliness, common repairs in the home, and equipment that can be helpful in maintaining a household).

Independent living skill units that are more complex and demand more from the client include management of funds and nutrition, food shopping, and meal preparation. Financial management covers areas such as budgeting, use of a bank account, investments, use of credit, and sources of financial assistance. Nutrition, food shopping, and meal preparation can begin with material such as the balanced diet, convenience foods, and selection of foods in stores, and progress to the specifics of meal preparation and use of kitchen utensils. Although all of the independent living skill units involve assignments and "in vivo" activities or homework, the financial management and nutrition sequence can require more practice activities than many of the others.

Two independent living skill units that should be emphasized are transportation and health care/medical management. Since many individuals are not seizure free and, based upon their state laws (see page 240), may be unable to secure a driver's license, understanding of different methods of transportation is a crucial step toward independent living. A transportation course includes how to use public transportation (bus, train, etc.), information on discounted transportation passes, cost comparisons of different transportation, securing emergency transportation, and so forth. In lieu of a driver's license, clients should be told how to obtain some sort of personal ID—for example, a passport.

For people with epilepsy, the value of a health care or medical management course in relation to the disability cannot be overemphasized. This course can involve an educational overview of epilepsy, but should also present specifics regarding medical resources in the community, techniques of ensuring appropriate medication compliance, recognition of medication side effects, aspects of health care insurance, resources for purchase of anticonvulsants less expensively, and steps to take in dealing with a seizure or an emergency situation. This health care course is extremely important for the young adult moving toward independence and can be a cornerstone to any independent living skills program.

Group Homes

In order to train persons with epilepsy in the skills of independent living, some epilepsy organizations have established group homes. A group home provides short-term residential facilities for a limited number of persons. Usually a resident staff member is on the premises at all times, and other staff members are on call to provide counseling or referral when necessary. Residents are generally instructed in financial management and housekeeping skills and are responsible for food shopping, cooking, cleaning up, and other household tasks.

A usual stipulation is that residents be employed or enrolled in a job-training program. Some group homes also require residents to be in therapy or counseling. Recreational opportunities are often provided at the home.

A group home can be a valuable "halfway house" for the person with epilepsy, providing an opportunity to learn independent living skills in a supportive environment. Unfortunately, the number of group homes now in existence is very limited.

ANTICONVULSANTS AND LIFE ADJUSTMENT

As persons with epilepsy begin making steps toward rehabilitation or independent living, it becomes important for an involved human services agency to determine the nature of their medical care. A person with an active seizure disorder should be seen by a neurologist every three to six months. The current practice is to work toward treatment with one primary anticonvulsant at a maximum tolerable dose. While it is sometimes necessary for a medical regimen to involve several anticonvulsants, this can lead to drug interactions that severely impair aspects of life performance. If a person requires several anticonvulsants to gain seizure control, administration of the new drugs should be monitored over a period of time to ensure therapeutic ranges and identify possible side effects. It becomes very important that the anticonvulsant blood serum levels taken by a hospital laboratory be of a reliable quality. Benchmarks in relation to quality blood serum testing can be the laboratory's participation in the Antiepileptic Drug Levels Quality Control Program at Columbia University in New York,[97] or the laboratory's use of gas liquid chromatography (GLC) or the Enzyme Multiple Immunoassay Technique (EMIT) for determining blood levels.[98]

The individual is often the prime determiner of whether the anticonvulsant program will be optimal. This involves not only compliance with the anticonvulsant regimen as prescribed, but also prompt reporting of any side effects and discussion with the neurologist of any over-the-counter drugs used. Many individuals with epilepsy fail to realize that their poor coordination, sleepiness, or, in fact, a depressive state can be related to anticonvulsant side effects. In other cases, a basic over-the-counter drug such as aspirin can interact with Dilantin, resulting in toxic effects from the Dilantin. Communication lines between patient and neurologist must be maintained.

LEGAL ASPECTS OF EPILEPSY

For decades, individuals with epilepsy have had basic rights violated in a number of areas. During the last several years, legislation such as the Education for All Handicapped Children Act of 1975 (P.L. 94-142) and the Developmental Disabilities Bill of Rights Act of 1975 (P.L.94-103) have established a number of specific rights for members of the population with epilepsy, along with those of other developmentally disabled groups. These rights include: individual education plans, the right to receive treatment in the least restrictive environment (i.e., alternatives to institutionalization), and gains in various areas related to personal (the right to marry) or community rights (the right to live in a residential community).

Common difficulties encountered by many individuals with epilepsy involve discrimination relating to employment and housing. In the area of employment, the job applicant with epilepsy must only inform the employer of the disability if it would affect performance of job duties (this, of course, may be done in the interview rather than on the application form). A discrimination suit may be initiated against an employer at any time, but it is important for the person with epilepsy to candidly assess skills, abilities, and safety factors in relation to the desired job. Similarly, an effort should be made to factually counter employer objections whenever possible (see pages 200-202).

In the job applicant's favor, it is important to realize that a business having a contract with the government for more than $2,500 must make "reasonable accommodation" to hire the handicapped (Section 503 of the Rehabilitation Act of 1973). "Reasonable accommodation" might involve restructuring parts of the job in order that dangerous conditions such as heights or exposure to molten liquids could be avoided for an active-seizure status person. A discrimination suit may be initiated against an employer through the Department of Labor's Office of Federal Contract Compliance or local equal or human rights offices at no cost to the claimant. In our experience, individuals who have won discrimination claims have encountered no repercussions once allowed onto the job.

Discrimination claims in relation to housing can also be initiated through local equal or human rights offices and tenants' associations. Tenants' associations can be very helpful in advising a person as to how to proceed when confronted with an apparent case of housing discrimination. In our Center's experience, housing discrimination issues are less frequent and have generally been settled without any legal action.

State laws vary in relation to a person with epilepsy being able to drive. In some states a seizure-free period of only six months is required, while in other states the period is two to three years. In some cases an appeal may be made to a state Department of Licensing (e.g., when individuals have infrequent partial motor seizures in which they are conscious and can pull off the road), with a license sometimes being granted. The success of these appeals can vary based upon the motorist's normal travel routes, the supporting physician's letter, and so forth. Concerns relating to automobile licensing are prevalent among the population with epilepsy.

The Developmentally Disabled Assistance and Bill of Rights Act (P.L. 95-

602) of 1978 defines a developmental disability as a severe, chronic disability related to a mental and/or physical impairment which is manifested before an individual reaches 22. As defined in this act, the developmental disability is likely to continue indefinitely and result in significant impediments to life functioning in three or more of the following areas: self-care, economic sufficiency, receptive and expressive language, mobility, capacity for independent living, learning, and self-direction.

This act mirrors the need for interdisciplinary treatment of extended duration that is crucial for many chronic seizure patients and those more severely impaired by other developmental disabilities. More specifically, local Developmental Disability Bureaus are responsible for case management services, child development services, alternative community living arrangement services, and nonvocational social development services. These services must be not only provided, but also detailed in an individually written habilitation plan. This act should further ensure better quality of services for the more severely impaired individual with epilepsy.

For a comprehensive and recent overview of more of the legal aspects of epilepsy, the reader is directed to the Epilepsy Foundation of America's new resource manual.[99] For a discussion of advocacy in relation to persons with epilepsy, see pages 250-51.

INSURANCE CONCERNS

Insurance coverage is frequently a major area of concern for people with epilepsy. Life insurance is generally easier to secure than other forms of insurance. Premiums can be similar to the non-disabled population or range up to several hundred percent higher. Life insurance can also be secured through the Epilepsy Foundation of America, which uses Government Employees' Life Insurance (GELI). The rates provided by this company approximate those of normal group rates. For many people with more severe forms of epilepsy, life insurance is still too costly or remains unavailable. As more precise actuarial data become available, there should be a continuing loosening of stringent coverage guidelines and reduction of life insurance costs.

Health insurance is more difficult to procure and is generally very costly. An individual who can receive group health (or life) insurance through a place of employment is generally choosing the best option. In large companies, group health insurance rates are simply based upon the sex and age characteristics of the company's employees. For those working in smaller companies, health expense claim experiences are usually pooled by the insurers among firms with less than 100 or less than 50 employees. In some cases, health insurance will not cover epilepsy-related treatment costs (considered a preexisting condition) for those working in smaller companies. If a person with epilepsy is self-employed or simply must seek an individual health insurance program, there are a number of insurance companies that will underwrite. More recently, several insurance companies (Prudential Insurance Company of America and Bankers Life and Casualty, Chicago) have reduced the extra health coverage premium for people with epilepsy.[100]

For any kind of insurance, especially health or automobile insurance, it is wise to compare costs and coverage among a number of companies. These rates may be changing dramatically over the next several years. Local epilepsy associations or a good insurance broker can assist in identifying a company with adequate coverage at reasonable costs. Premiums will, of course, vary with the experience of the various insurance companies.

MALE-FEMALE RELATIONSHIPS AND MARRIAGE CONCERNS

When one considers the dependency and social isolation fostered by epilepsy, it becomes obvious that social deficits may impede the development of normal male-female relationships. In a study by Edwards,[101] 58 percent of his sample (n = 166) complained that their social lives had been restricted by the disability, and 46 percent of marriageable age had never married. People with epilepsy should be encouraged by parents and significant others to mix with members of the opposite sex. Learning to discuss seizures or accept a seizure occurrence when accompanied by a member of the opposite sex can become real social turning points. Involvement in a social skills program, such as the previously discussed Human Relationships and Sexuality class (see page 209), can serve both an informative and supportive function for adults with epilepsy.

In approaching marriage, a frequent concern of the adult with epilepsy is the role of heredity in relation to a son or daughter having epilepsy. If one parent has epilepsy, there appears to be minimal risk that a son or daughter will develop seizures, but it can be wise to consult a neurologist or genetic counselor. See pages 50-54 for a discussion of this matter.

EPILEPSY AND EXERCISE

Involvement in some type of physical exercise or formal sports program is generally to be encouraged for people with epilepsy. This type of activity not only improves physical conditioning and performance skills, but can generalize so that the person develops a higher level of self-confidence and better capabilities for handling stress. Team sports can foster interpersonal skills and the ability to cooperate in pursuit of a common goal—valuable assets in later life. Results from a parent survey completed in the Northeast[102] indicated that children with epilepsy participated more often in sports than in any of the other leisure time activities mentioned.

Kuijer[103] recently completed a study on epilepsy and exercise involving young adults with an active seizure status at the Heemstede Center in Holland. Methods involved a comparison of the effects of continuous (215 trials) versus intermittent (230 trials) stationary bicycle exercise. The duration of each bicycle trial was 45 minutes. Results indicate that only one seizure was observed during all trials of either type of exercise; but in the period immediately following the exercise program, 128 seizures were recorded for the continuous exercise group and 27 for those who had been involved in the intermittent exercise. Results suggest that the person with epilepsy should take basic precautions during the period immediately following exercise, and that brief periods of exercise coupled with intermittent rest (for example, simply walking) seem to reduce the probability of having a seizure later. Less strenuous exercise would also reduce the likelihood of seizures.

For those with more severe forms of epilepsy and associated disabilities, exercise programs that can be performed while sitting in a chair (such as those recommended by various airlines) can be utilized. The Day Care Center in Hvidovre, Denmark, has used this type of program as well as a formal gymnasium physical education program for those with severe seizure conditions.[104] In the case of a gymnasium program, the attendance of several staff members is recommended when working with a severely seizure-impaired group.

CONCLUSIONS

This chapter has outlined some of the major areas of life adjustment difficulties for the person with epilepsy and has offered rehabilitation or habilitation approaches that can be used to counter problems within these areas. There are, of course, a number of people with epilepsy who will not encounter significant vocational, social, or independent living difficulties. Unfortunately, though, among the chronic seizure patients and those with associated disabilities who are served at our centers and rehabilitation facilities, these difficulties will be prevalent. Nevertheless, through the efforts of medical and human service professionals both in our country and abroad, improved services continue to be developed and more comprehensive plans initiated to engage the identified problems.

REFERENCES

1. Rodin, E.A., Shapiro, H.L. and Lennox, K.: Epilepsy and life performance. *Rehabilitation Literature,* 38: 34-38, 1977.
2. Ibid, p. 38.
3. Rehabilitation Services Administration (University of Florida Rehabilitation Research Institute, Gainsville). Transitional employment enhances job placement for epileptic clients. *Rehabilitation Brief,* 4, 1978.
4. Epilepsy Foundation of America. *Basic Statistics on the Epilepsies.* Philadelphia: F.A. Davis, 1975.
5. Emlen, A.C. and Ryan, R.: Analyzing unemployment rates among men with epilepsy. In preparation.
6. Ibid.
7. Rodin, E., Rennick, P., Dennerll, R. and Lin, Y.: Vocational and educational problems of epileptic patients. *Epilepsia,* 13: 149-160, 1972.
8. Farrago, F.: Disability in epileptics. *Epilepsia,* 13: 63-70, 1972.
9. Perlman, L.G.: *The Person with Epilepsy: Lifestyle, Needs, Expectations.* Chicago: National Epilepsy League, 1977. (A "needs assessment" survey of the National Epilepsy League's clients.)
10. Fraser, R., Erikson, K. and Thompson, J.: The role of specialized vocational services in comprehensive treatment of the individual with epilepsy. Paper presented at the Epilepsy International Symposium, Vancouver, B.C., Canada, September 1978. Arlington, Va.: Eric Microfilm No. Ed 168 267, 1978.
11. Epilepsy Foundation of America, 1975, op. cit.
12. Rodin, E.A.: Medical and social prognosis in epilepsy. *Epilepsia,* 13: 121-131, 1972.
13. Epi-Hab Phoenix, Inc., Arizona. *A Project to Determine the Employability of Epileptics.* Final report, SRS grant PB-214-225, 1971.
14. Risch, F.: We lost every game . . . but. *Rehabilitation Record,* 9: 16-18, 1968.
15. Kuijer, A.: *Epilepsy and Exercise.* "Meer En Bosch" Heemstede, Netherlands: S.R.A.E., 1978. (Available from Dr. Kuijer, c/o Stichting Kempenhaeghe, Sterkseleweg 65, Heeze, N.B., Netherlands.)
16. Epilepsy Foundation of America, 1975, op. cit.
17. Wright, G.N. (ed.): *Epilepsy Rehabilitation.* Boston: Little, Brown, 1975.
18. Fraser, R. et al., 1978, op. cit.
19. Frank, D.S.: Group counseling benefits job seekers with epilepsy. *Rehabilitation Record,* 9: 34-37, 1968.
20. Schlesinger, L.E. and Frank, D.: From demonstration to dissemination: Gateways to employment for epileptics. *Rehabilitation Literature,* 35: 98-106, 109, 1974.
21. Testing materials and scoring services available from Interpretive Scoring Systems, 4401 W. 76th Street, Minneapolis, MN 55435.
22. Testing materials and scoring services available from Science Research Associates, Inc., 259 E. Erie Street, Chicago, IL 60611.
23. Available from the Psychological Corporation, 757 Third Avenue, New York, NY 10017.
24. Available from the American Association on Mental Deficiency, 5201 Connecticut Avenue, N.W., Washington, DC 20015.
25. Danielsen, J. and Petersen, V.: The frequency of subclinical absences in patients with epilepsy and in children with school trouble. *Electroencephalography and Clinical Neurophysiology,* 43: 518-519, 1977.
26. Reitan, R.M.: A research program on the psychological effects of brain lesions in human beings. In: N.R. Ellis (ed.), *International Review of Research in Mental Retardation,* Vol. 1. New York: Academic Press, 1966.
27. Dodrill, C.B.: A neuropsychological battery for epilepsy. *Epilepsia,* 19: 611-623, 1978.
28. U.S. Department of Labor, Manpower Administration. *Vocational Exploration Group: Theory and Research,* prepared by Calvin J. Daane. Washington, DC: U.S. Government Printing Office, 1972.
29. Daane, C.J.: Job personalization and the vocational exploration group. *Journal of Employment Counseling,* 10: 3-10, 1973.
30. Anderson, J.A.: The disadvantaged see work through their efforts or ours? *Rehabilitation Record,* 9: 5-10, 1968.
31. Azrin, N.H., Flores, T. and Kaplan, S.J.: Job-finding club: A group-assisted program for obtaining employment. *Behavior Research and Therapy,* 13: 17-27, 1975.

32. Sutton, D., Smith, W.R. and Fraser, R.T.: A comparative study of parent counseling approaches. Paper presented at the Thirtieth Annual Western Institute on Epilepsy, Portland, OR, March 1979.
33. Hicks, R.A. and Hicks, M.J.: Changes over a 10-year period (1956–1966) in the employer's attitudes towards the employment of epileptics. *American Corrective Therapy Journal*, 22: 145-147, 1968.
34. Barrow, R.: *Epilepsy and the Law*. 2nd ed. New York: Harper & Row, 1966.
35. Sands, H. and Zalkind, S.S.: Effects of an educational campaign to change employer attitudes toward hiring epileptics. *Epilepsia*, 13: 87-96, 1972.
36. Fraser, R., Trejo, W., Dikmen, S. and Temkin, N.: Changing employer attitudes towards hiring those with epilepsy. In preparation.
37. Zielinski, J.J.: Social prognosis in epilepsy. *Epilepsia*, 13: 133-140, 1972.
38. Horten, J. TAPS project coordinator, 1017 N. Main Street, Suite 220, San Antonio, Texas 78212. Personal communication.
39. Hicks, R.A. and Hicks, M.J., 1968, op. cit.
40. Epi-Hab Phoenix, Inc., 1971, op. cit.
41. Risch, F., 1968, op. cit.
42. Sands, H.: Report of a study undertaken for the Committee on Neurological Disorders in Industry. Council on Industrial Health, American Medical Association. Abstracted in *Epilepsy News*, 7, 1961.
43. Epilepsy Foundation of America. *New Directions in Epilepsy Rehabilitation: A Resource Manual*. Washington, D.C.: 1979.
44. Sinick, D.: Job placement and post-placement services for the epileptic client. In: G.N. Wright (ed.) *Epilepsy Rehabilitation*. Boston: Little, Brown, 1975.
45. Perlman, L.G., 1977, op. cit., p. 31.
46. Fraser, R. et al., 1978, op. cit.
47. Sands, H. and Radin, J.: *The Mentally Disabled Rehabilitant: Post-Employment Services*. RSA grant 15-P-59135/2-01. 2nd ed. New York: Postgraduate Center for Mental Health, 1979.
48. Dennerll, R.D., Rodin, E.A., Gonzalez, S., Schwartz, M.L. and Lin, T.: Neurological and psychological factors related to employability of persons with epilepsy. *Epilepsia*, 7: 318-319, 1966.
49. Krohn, W.: A study of epilepsy in northern Norway, its frequency and character. *Acta Psychiatrica Neurologica Scandinavica* (Supplement 150) 36: 215-225, 1961.
50. Rodin, E., et al., 1972, op. cit.
51. Scott, D.F.: Review article: Psychiatric aspects of epilepsy. *British Journal of Psychiatry*, 132: 417-430, 1978.
52. Betts, T.A., Mersky, H. and Pond, D.A.: Psychiatry. In: J. Lindlaw and A. Richens (eds.) *A Textbook of Epilepsy*. Edinburgh: Churchill Livingston, 1976.
53. Bagley, C.: *The Social Psychology of the Child with Epilepsy*. London: Routledge and Kegan Paul, 1971.
54. Bear, D.M. and Fedio, P.: Quantitative analysis of interictal behavior in temporal lobe epilepsy. *Archives of Neurology*, 34: 454-476, 1977.
55. Pond, D.A. and Bidwell, B.H.: A Survey of epilepsy in 14 general practices. II Social and psychological aspects. *Epilepsia*, 1: 285, 1959.
56. Taylor, D.C.: Psychiatry and sociology in the understanding of epilepsy. B.M. Mandelbrae and M.J. Golden (eds.), *Psychiatric Aspects of Medical Practice*. London: Staples Press, 1972.
57. Rutter, M., Graham, P. and Yule, W.: *A Neuropsychiatric Study in Childhood*. Lavenham, Suffolk: Lavenham Press, 1970.
58. Bakker, C.G. and Armstrong, H.E.: Implementation of an educational approach to the delivery of mental health services. *Hospital and Community Psychiatry* 27: 330-334, 1976.
59. Hersen, M. and Bellack, A.G.: Social skills training for chronic patients: Rationale, research, findings, and future directions. *Comprehensive Psychiatry* 17: 559-580, 1976.
60. Goldsmith, J.B. and McFall, R.M.: Development and evaluation of an interpersonal skill training program for psychiatric inpatients. *Journal of Abnormal Psychology* 84: 51-58, 1975.
61. Mitchell, K.R. and White, R.G.: Behavioral self-management: An application to the problem of migraine headaches. *Behavior Therapy* 8: 213-221, 1977.
62. Rehm, L.P. and Marston, A.R.: Reduction of social anxiety through modification of self-reinforcement: An instigation therapy technique. *Journal of Consulting and Clinical Psy-*

chology 32: 565-574, 1968.
63. Mostofsky, D. and Balasbak, B.I.: Psychobiological control of seizures. *Psychological Bulletin* 84: 723-750, 1977.
64. Parrino, J.J.: Reduction of seizures by desensitization. *Journal of Behavior Therapy and Experimental Psychiatry* 2: 215-218, 1971.
65. Wells, K.C., Turner, S.M., Bellack, A.S. and Hersen, M.: Effects of cue-controlled relaxation on psychomotor seizures: An experimental analysis. *Behavior Research and Therapy* 16: 51-53, 1978.
66. Zlutnick, S., Mayville, W.J. and Moffot, S.: Modification of seizure disorders: The interruption of behavioral chains. *Journal of Applied Behavior Analysis* 8: 1-12, 1975.
67. Seligman, M.E.P.: *Helplessness: On Depression, Development, and Death*. San Francisco: Freeman, 1975.
68. Brulleman, L.H.: Group therapy with epileptic patients at the Instituut voor Epilepsie-bestrijding. *Epilepsia* 13: 225-231, 1972.
69. Lessman, S.E. and Mollick, L.R.: Group treatment of epileptics. *Health and Social Work* 3: 106-121, 1978.
70. Mayer, B. and Gutjahr, L.: Pilot study on theme-centered interaction groups with epileptic patients. In: J.K. Penry (ed.), *Epilepsy, The Eighth International Symposium*. New York: Raven Press, 1977.
71. Scarborough, L.F.: Management of convulsive patients by group therapy. *Diseases of the Nervous System* 17: 223, 1956.
72. McFall, R.M. and Marston, A.R.: An experimental investigation of behavior rehearsal in assertive training. *Journal of Abnormal Psychology* 76: 295-303, 1970.
73. McFall, R.M. and Twentyman, C.T.: Four experiments on the relative contributions of rehearsal, modeling, and coaching to assertive training. *Journal of Abnormal Psychology* 81: 199-218, 1973.
74. Bernstein, D.A. and Borkovec, T.D.: *Progressive Relaxation Training: A Manual for the Helping Professions*. Champaign, IL: Research Press, 1973.
75. Lubar, J.F.: Clinical applications of EEG feedback, including treatment of epilepsy. Presentation at Biomedical Services Incorporated, Clinical Biofeedback Seminar, San Francisco, September, 1978.
76. Galassi, J.P., Galassi, M.D. and Litz, M.C.: Assertive training in groups using video feedback. *Journal of Counseling Psychology*, 21: 390-394, 1974.
77. Lamont, J.F., Gilner, F.H., Spector, N.G. and Skinner, K.K.: Group Assertion Training and Group Insight Therapies. *Psychological Reports* 25: 463-470, 1969.
78. Lange, A.J. and Jakobowski, P.: *Responsible Assertive Behavior: Cognitive/Behavioral Procedures for Trainers*. Champaign, IL: Research Press, 1976.
79. Lewinsohn, P.M. and Graf, M.: Placement activities and depression. *Journal of Consulting and Clinical Psychology* 41: 261-268, 1973.
80. Meichenbaum, D.H.: *Cognitive Behavior Modifications*. New York: Plenum, 1977.
81. Dikmen, S., Matthews, C.G. and Harley, J.P.: Effect of early versus late onset of major motor epilepsy on cognitive-intellectual performance: Further considerations. *Epilepsia* 18: 31-36, 1977.
82. Treat, N.J., Poon, L.W., Fozard, J.L. and Popkin, S.J.: Toward applying cognitive skill training to memory problems. Paper presented at the Annual Convention of the American Psychological Association, San Francisco, 1977.
83. Chapman, L.F. and Wolf, H.G.: The cerebral hemisphere and the highest integrative functions of man. *A.M.A. Archives of Neurology*, 1: 357-424, 1959.
84. D'Zurilla, T.J. and Goldfried, M.R.: Problem-solving and behavior modification. *Journal of Abnormal Behavior* 78: 107-126, 1971.
85. Goldfried, M.R. and Davison, G.C.: Problem-solving, In: *Clinical Behavior Therapy*. New York: Holt, Rinehart & Winston, 1976.
86. Smith, W.R. and Queisser, H.R.: Group training in problem-solving skills for patients with epilepsy. Paper presented at the Epilepsy International Symposium, Vancouver, B.C., Canada, September, 1978.
87. Smith, W.R. and Queisser, H.R.: Group training in problem-solving skills in epilepsy rehabilitation. Unpublished manuscript, University of Washington Epilepsy Center, Seattle, 1979.
88. Kühlman, A. director, Day Care Center, Karetmagerporten 3A, 2650 Hvidovre, Denmark. Personal communication.

89. McFall, R.M. Parameters of self-monitoring. In: R.B. Stuart (ed.), *Behavioral Self-Management: Strategies, Techniques, and Outcomes*. New York: Brunner/Mazel, 1977.
90. Sutton, D. et al., 1979, op. cit.
91. Walton, K.M., Schwab, L.O., Cassett-Dunn, M.A. and Wright, V.K.: Independent living techniques and concepts: Level of use vs. importance to independent living as perceived by professionals in rehabilitation. Department Report 2, RSA Grant 44-P-81256/7-01, University of Nebraska Department of Human Development and the Family College of Home Economics, 1968.
92. Krantz, G.: Critical vocational behaviors. *Journal of Rehabilitation*, 37: 14-16, 1971.
93. Sutton, D. et al., 1979, op. cit.
94. Hartlage, L.C., Green, J.B. and Offutt, L.: Dependency in epileptic children. *Epilepsia*, 13: 27-30, 1972.
95. Lund, M. and Randrup, J.: A day-centre for severely handicapped people with epilepsy. *Epilepsia* 13: 245-247, 1972.
96. Sergesketter, C. vocational evaluator, Tri-State Epilepsy Association, Inc., 421 North Main Street, Evansville, Indiana. Personal communication.
97. List of participating laboratories available from Dr. Charles Pippenger, Box 90, Neurological Institute, 710 W. 168 Street, New York, NY 10032.
98. Levine, I. Getting to know the epilepsies, *Patient Care*, 11: 102-136, 1977.
99. Epilepsy Foundation of America, 1979, op. cit.
100. McAllister, J. executive director, Epilepsy Foundation of America. Memo dated May 31, 1979.
101. Edwards, V.E.: Social problems confronting a person with epilepsy in modern society. *Proceedings of the Australian Association of Neurologists* 11: 239-243, 1974.
102. Goldin, G.J., Perry, S.L., Margolin, R.J., Stotsky, B.A. and Foster, J.C.: *Rehabilitation of the Young Epileptic*. Lexington, MA: D.C. Heath, 1977.
103. Kuijer, A., personal communication, op. cit.
104. Kühlman, A., personal communication, op. cit.

IV.
HELPING RESOURCES

9

RESOURCES FOR EPILEPSY: ACCESS AND ADVOCACY

RISHA W. LEVINSON, D.S.W.

All people have difficulties in locating services to meet their many needs, and so do persons with epilepsy. While there is a proliferation of health and social services and a considerable wealth of information in published materials, the actual linking of the person with epilepsy with an appropriate, available, and accessible service often presents overwhelming problems for the provider as well as for the consumer. In addition to the usual barriers in locating services, as well as persistent negative societal attitudes, recognition must also be given to the idiosyncratic nature of epilepsy itself, including the medical and social implications associated with this disorder.

According to the dictionary definition, access is "the right to enter or make use of," which implies a universal, equitable, barrier-free entry to all human resources, as well as the opportunity to use these resources as needed. Yet, for persons (and families) concerned with epilepsy, gaining access is often difficult.

BARRIERS TO SERVICES

Barriers in reaching needed services are encountered by everyone. Discrimination, lack of adequate transportation, gas cost and shortages, inconvenient hours of services, problems of eligibility, inaccessibility of location, financial restrictions, and problems of language and communication are but a few of the many roadblocks that hamper connections with existing services.

The author acknowledges with thanks the generous assistance of the following staff members of the Epilepsy Foundation of America: Susan Ames, Alexandra K. Finucan, Suzanne Fulton, Melinda Hatton, and Nyrma Hernandez.

These impediments present problems for the poor, the elderly, ethnic and minority groups, but particularly for the disabled.

It is well known that individuals with epilepsy find employment more difficult to procure, since many employers are hesitant to hire them. Educational opportunities are less readily available, and recreational activities may not welcome the person with epilepsy. In short, biases toward those with epilepsy still exist.

Given that epilepsy is for many persons a lifelong condition, access to services should ideally fit into a total life plan within the phases of the human life cycle. However, current realities reflect a disjointed, fragmented, and uncoordinated system of services.

It has been observed that "to be a person with a handicapping condition requiring a range of activities over a prolonged period of time is like being a pinball in a pinball machine. One is bounced hither and yon—sometimes scoring very well, and other times missing the mark and falling back into the return slot, only to be bounced around again at some future time."[1]

Despite the multitude and range of health and social services that exist, no centralized source for information and referral to human resources is currently available, nor is there a centralized information and data base on epilepsy in particular. Then how can access be facilitated within some system of accountability to document what services there are? How can the consumer best be linked with what services, and with what outcome?

ACCESS TO SERVICES

The decade of the 1960s ushered in an era of consumerism and a demand for the right to access, which sparked off the development of Information and Referral Services, generally referred to as "I & R" (see pages 241-42). During the past two decades, I & R services have proliferated in many public and voluntary agencies, supported by growing numbers of service organizations and consumer groups. Since the 1965 legislation of the Older Americans Act, the Administration on Aging has mandated programs in many community and state agencies. Title XX Social Services monies have, since 1975, also contributed to the development of state and local systems of I & R by designating this as a universal service, to be made available to all citizens, irrespective of age, status, or income.

A review of the current state of the art in I & R programs reveals an impressive development of growing numbers of sophisticated manual and computerized programs that aim to standardize human information systems and to arrive at uniform I & R reporting procedures.[2]

In many directories of services, I & R is listed as an auxiliary service or as a single agency function within a multifunctional service agency. However, an Information and Referral program is to be regarded as a service modality as well as an ongoing process. This process entails giving information through an organized resource-information system (operative through manual or computerized operations), following up referrals within a system of accountability, and assuming the advocacy role. The information (I), referral (R), and advocacy (A) components constitute a proposed access system, identified with the acronym IRA.

OVERVIEW OF SELECTED SERVICES AND RESOURCES

This chapter is directed primarily to the service provider who has the responsibility of responding to inquiries for information, giving advice, offering counseling, and, where indicated, making referral to other resources. To be an effective helper, the provider needs to have a knowledge of the disorder of epilepsy and a familiarity with the major programs, organizations, and services available to persons with epilepsy.

Thus, in the following sections we shall discuss medical and dental care; insurance; financial assistance; employment and vocational rehabilitation; education; housing; transportation; and personal social services. For further follow-up on information, and/or advocacy action, the official titles and address of service programs and service organizations are listed on pages 253-57.

MEDICAL AND DENTAL CARE AND MEDICAL ASSISTANCE

It has been noted that for people with epilepsy the greatest hope is to be free of seizures. Intervention at an early stage can reduce seizures and actually be a preventive measure. Many problems associated with patient compliance with a medication regime can be attributed to lack of continuous and consistent medical care. Lack of knowledge of the need for continued care, inaccessibility of physicians and clinics, and high expenses entailed in securing medical treatment are some of the major reasons why adequate medical attention is not secured by many persons with epilepsy. The high cost of anticonvulsant medication is also a deterring factor.

It is critically important that children receive early diagnosis, medical care, and preventive treatment since a large percentage of epilepsy cases develop before the age of 20 (see Chapter 7). If a family does not know where to turn for information on epilepsy and referral to a primary care physician or specialist (pediatrician, neurologist, epileptologist), undue time, effort, and money may be spent in wasteful "doctor shopping," which delays appropriate treatment and provokes anxieties.

As for dental care, it is important to receive the treatment for special dental problems that may be encountered by persons with epilepsy, including fractured teeth and broken jaws sustained when a seizure episode was mishandled by having a hard object forced between the teeth, or gum conditions that may be linked to anticonvulsant medication (see page 37).

Following is an overview of selected medical and dental services. Further information can be obtained from the local chapters or state and national offices of the Epilepsy Foundation of America.

Referral Sources: Medical and Dental Care

Physicians and Dentists. Referral for medical and dental practitioners and specialists is generally available through their professional organizations, the American Medical Association and the American Dental Association.

Clinics. Information on clinics is included in the most recent *Guide to Epilepsy* (1978) published by the Epilepsy Foundation of America. This guide is an update of the list of clinics included in the 1973 publication by EFA.

EFA Low-Cost Drug Program. This low-cost drug program is available to all members of the Epilepsy Foundation of America and their immediate families. Members may send their doctors' prescriptions to the Prescription Delivery System in Hatboro, Pennsylvania, where prescriptions are usually filled in about 96 hours and mailed to the client by first class mail. A price list can be obtained by writing to the pharmacy service directly.

Epilepsy Research Centers. Under the Public Health Services Act (P.L. 94-63, Section 604), the Epilepsy Branch of the National Institute of Neurological and Communicative Disorders and Stroke (NINCDS) operates Epilepsy Research Centers (Comprehensive Epilepsy Programs) located in the states of California, Georgia, Minnesota, Oregon, Virginia, Washington, Michigan, North Carolina, South Carolina, and Tennessee. These programs are designed to facilitate clinical research and to coordinate research and teaching within a defined geographic area. Programs are expected to serve as models for research and are designed to explore new means for effective health service delivery to those with epilepsy.

Referral Sources: Medical Assistance

The primary sources of federal medical assistance for aged and/or indigent disabled persons are Medicare and Medicaid. Special programs for children include the Early Periodic Screening, Diagnosis, and Treatment Program, and the Crippled Children's Services.

Medicare. This health insurance program under Social Security is designed to serve everyone over 65 years of age and also disabled persons under 65 years of age who have been entitled to receive Social Security benefits or railroad disability annuities for two consecutive years or more, and who need dialysis treatment or a kidney transplant because of permanent kidney failure. The program is not based on income, but is available regardless of financial need.

The Medicare program has two parts. Part A provides hospital insurance at no cost to pay for care while in the hospital and for selected health care services after leaving the hospital. Part B provides voluntary medical insurance for a relatively low monthly charge that helps pay doctor bills and other approved medical services.

More information about Medicare is available from the local Social Security office, or by writing to the designated federal agency.

Medicaid. Medicaid (Medical Assistance Programs) is a joint federal/state program to provide physical and related health care services to persons with low incomes. Disabled persons may be eligible for Medicaid on the basis of income. Because eligibility is determined by the individual state's program of public assistance (welfare) on the basis of broad federal guidelines, there are geographic differences between eligibility requirements and types of services covered. Generally, persons may be eligible for Medicaid if they are receiving welfare, other public assistance benefits, or Supplemental Security Income (SSI). Medicaid services are available in all states except Arizona.

Each state has the option of providing individuals or their children with Medicaid services if medical expenses exceed a given percentage of their annual income.

Further information and application for Medicaid is available at local or state welfare or public assistance offices. If local information cannot be obtained, inquire at the designated federal agency.

Crippled Children's Services (CCS). Crippled Children's Services is a joint federal/state program to provide medical and related services to handicapped children from birth to age 21. This program is included under Title V of the Social Security Act, which authorizes formula grants to states for Maternal and Child Health and Crippled Children's Services. The program has significance for diagnosis and treatment services for low-income expectant mothers with epilepsy.

Title V also provides for the training of health personnel from many disciplines to work with handicapped and retarded children in 20 University-Affiliated Facility (UAF) programs.

It is important to note that states are free to determine the kinds of services and disabling conditions they will serve within their respective programs for

Crippled Children's Services. No state residency period is generally required before such services are provided. The range and cost of additional treatment or hospital care services varies from state to state. All programs accept third party payments, including Medicaid, Blue Cross and Blue Shield, and other medical insurance.

Further information is available at the local, county, or state health department.

Early Periodic Screening, Diagnosis, and Treatment Program (EPSDT). The EPSDT program screens children from poor families to identify whether health care or related services may be necessary. This program has the potential of case-finding and assuring follow-up, with appropriate linkage to needed services, thereby promoting seizure control at an early age. Children receiving state Aid to Families of Dependent Children benefits and children whose parents or guardians are receiving Medicaid and/or local or state public assistance benefits are eligible for EPSDT. EPSDT programs vary from state to state and are administered by either state departments of social services or by health departments.

More information on EPSDT is available from the local or state health department or public assistance office.

LIFE INSURANCE

Obtaining adequate insurance coverage at reasonable rates has been a serious problem for many persons with epilepsy, particularly for applicants having more than one grand mal or petit mal attack per year.

The Epilepsy Foundation of America offers group life insurance policies for those with epilepsy who are employed at least 20 hours a week "and do not have a life-threatening disease." Eligibility is determined by the insurance company from confidential application information.[3]

The EFA Group Plan is underwritten by Government Employees Life Insurance Co. of Washington, D.C., and applications are processed through the Epilepsy Foundation of America.

TAX BENEFITS

In computing income tax due, the Internal Revenue Service allows medical and dental expenses to be deducted from earned income (in this case, of the disabled individual or of his or her parents). Deductible items include special equipment and payments to a special school for a mentally or physically handicapped individual, if the principal reason for attendance is the institution's resources for alleviating the handicap. However, under the Education for All Handicapped Children Act of 1975 (P.L. 94-142), which is based on the principle of "mainstreaming," children may be placed in special schools or special classes "only when the nature or severity of the handicap is such that education in regular classes . . . cannot be achieved satisfactorily."

In addition, the IRS allows tax credits for the cost of disabled dependent or disabled spouse care. Payments to relatives who provide this care can be included in some circumstances.[4] Further information on tax credits and educations can be obtained from the local IRS office.

FINANCIAL ASSISTANCE

There are two basic federal programs providing direct and continuing financial assistance to disabled persons: Social Security Disability Insurance (DI) and Social Security Income (SSI).

Social Security Disability Insurance Benefits

Social Security Disability Insurance benefits (DI) provide continuing monthly income when individuals are unable to engage in "substantial gainful activity" (SGA) because they are disabled. SGA is defined in specific dollar amounts by the Social Security Administration. The upper limit for eligibility under the rules for determining "SGA" is $481, the level currently applied to the blind and the aged.

Persons may be considered disabled under this program if they "have a physical or mental impairment which prevents them from working; is expected to last, or has lasted, for at least 12 months, or is expected to result in death."

Two types of DI benefits are available: 1. Benefits for persons disabled since childhood are available if parents or guardians have paid in to Social Security during their work lives; and 2. benefits for persons disabled as adults are available through their own personal Social Security contributions when they were in the work force. If disabled before age 31, the individual needs one-and-a-half years of Social Security work credit to receive assistance. Eligibility for Disability Insurance automatically entitles the individual to Medicare.

Monthly benefits may be paid to disabled workers under 65 and their families. Disabled spouses, disabled dependent spouses, and, under some conditions, disabled surviving divorced spouses of workers who were insured at death may receive benefits at age 50 in these instances. If persons are disabled before age 22 and continue to be permanently disabled, benefits will last a lifetime and will continue after the death of parents. The parent who has personal responsibility for caring for the disabled dependent adult may also qualify for benefits.

The local Social Security office has many helpful booklets on benefits. Publications are available in English and Spanish and in Braille. Information concerning Social Security programs can be provided by the Social Security or Medicare number listed in the local telephone directory.

Supplemental Security Income (SSI)

Persons who are disabled and whose income and resources are very limited may be eligible for Supplemental Security Income benefits (Amendment to the Social Security Act, 1974). SSI is designed to provide a minimum monthly income for those whose disability prevents them from gainful employment and who, because of their disability, may not have been able to contribute to the regular Social Security system. Financial eligibility for SSI may be complex. It depends on a variety of factors, including living arrangements, savings, and assets.

To counteract the work disincentives that were formerly built into the Social Security Disability Insurance and the Supplemental Security Income legislation, the new Social Security Disability Amendments of 1980 tend to encourage entry and/or reentry into the work force with less risk of losing benefits.

In effect, the new law makes it less risky for people receiving financial assistance to see whether they can be gainfully employed. For example, the 1980 Amendments extend the trial work period and establish a formula for the gradual reduction of benefits. This legislation also provides for an experimental program which allows severely disabled persons with epilepsy to retain eligibility for important medical and social services beyond the income cut-off point. If the disability turns out to be too severe for work, or the job terminates, a second 24-month waiting period for benefits is eliminated.

In accordance with the Amendments of 1980, people with epilepsy who are receiving SSI and/or DI are allowed to deduct the costs of medication and services necessary to control their seizures from other income before that income is assessed for eligibility.

SSI may also be available to disabled children. If a person is under 18 years of age, not married, and not the head of a household, he or she is considered a "child" under SSI. Also, a disabled person is considered a child and therefore eligible for SSI if he or she is attending school on a full-time basis and is not more than 18 years of age.

The SSI program is important to people with low incomes who have epilepsy since other services are available to the SSI recipient—Medicaid, health services, vocational rehabilitation, social services, and food stamps.

Further information concerning possible income assistance is available from the district Social Security office.

EMPLOYMENT AND VOCATIONAL REHABILITATION

Despite the dramatic advances in the treatment and rehabilitation of epilepsy, and despite the federal legislation that prohibits discrimination against the handicapped, unemployment and underemployment are serious problems (see Chapter 8). Among the many factors which exacerbate this situation are the continued reluctance of employers to hire individuals with epilepsy, and the insecurity on the part of the employee who is faced with the dilemma of whether or not to conceal the condition of epilepsy. Other significant factors include lack of transportation to work for non-drivers and concerns over an unregulated medication schedule.

Job Placement

Helping handicapped job seekers is a specific responsibility of the more than 2,400 local Employment Security offices located throughout the United States. More commonly referred to as State Employment Service or State Job Service, these public employment centers are mandated by law to employ a specialist who is trained to work with disabled people in job placement or to refer the disabled person to another agency for further assistance.

Federal Job Opportunities

While most federal jobs are filled on a competitive basis, there are a small number of special "A" appointment positions for handicapped individuals. These jobs are not competitive and are available through the referral of a vocational rehabilitation counselor or by accepting a 700-hour trial appointment.

Additional federal employment possibilities are available through the Federal Job Information Centers, which are maintained by the U.S. Office of Personnel Management. Special arrangements for handicapped individuals are made by selected placement coordinators located in these Job Information Centers, generally listed under *U.S. Government* in local telephone directories.

Further information can be obtained by dialing 800/555-1212 for the toll-free number of a federal Job Information Center in a particular state.

The Comprehensive Employment and Training Program (CETA)

CETA was created to provide employment and training for the unemployed and underemployed, as well as the disabled and economically disadvantaged.

Contact the local State Employment Security Office of the mayor's office for more information about available CETA programs.

The Training and Placement Service (TAPS)

TAPS is administered through the Epilepsy Foundation of America and is funded under the CETA program by the United States Department of Labor.

The purpose of TAPS is to increase the employment rate of persons with epilepsy by providing support services and on-the-job training. TAPS services are aimed to assist people to get and maintain appropriate long-term employment. Both the employer and the client-employee benefit from the services provided by TAPS. For the employer, TAPS provides prospective employees who have received vocational training and furnishes on-the-job training funds. For the client-employee, TAPS offers vocational counseling, job-seeking skills training, work support groups, and placement assistance. Education services are offered to both employers and client-employees to promote a better understanding of the employment aspects of epilepsy.

In addition to the two national TAPS units located in the Epilepsy Foundation office in Washington D.C., TAPS services are available at training and placement project offices (in Atlanta, Georgia; Boston, Massachusetts; Cleveland, Ohio; Minneapolis, Minnesota; Portland, Oregon; and Bayamon, Puerto Rico) and satellite offices (in Lexington, Kentucky; New Orleans, Louisiana; Baltimore, Maryland; Duluth, Minnesota; and Charlotte, North Carolina). In addition, there are 11 TAPS-like employment programs that are grant-funded in Orlando, Florida; Boise, Lewiston, and Pocatello, Idaho; Rockford, Illinois; Worcester, Massachusetts; Jackson, Mississippi; Utica, New York; Knoxville and Memphis, Tennessee; and Richmond, Virginia.

Further information regarding the TAPS Programs is available at the National Office of the Epilepsy Foundation of America, Washington, D.C.

Small Business Administration (SBA)

Handicapped persons interested in going into business for themselves may qualify for federal assistance and low-cost loans from the national and state offices of the Small Business Administration.

Projects with Industry (PWI)

Several projects in which industry has been directly involved with efforts to place handicapped individuals have demonstrated favorable experiences. These projects, which represent opportunities to overcome reluctance in hiring persons with epilepsy, are currently under the auspices of the Administration of Developmental Disabilities, part of the Department of Education.

The 11-model Projects with Industry (PWI) are federally funded to place handicapped people in competitive jobs and involve company coordinators in the rehabilitation process. PWI has achieved a higher placement rate at less than half of the usual cost, and has identified new job opportunities.

Sheltered Workshops

The federal government provides financial support for sheltered employment, generally through state allocations. For some, these workshops may be preparation for reentry into a competitive work situation; for others, they may provide a lifetime work situation. The experience at Epi-Habs—nonprofit corporations that hire handicapped people in a sheltered setting—has been highly favorable, since it has demonstrated that many handicapped persons with epilepsy can perform effectively in an environment similar to that of industry.

Vocational Rehabilitation

All states have vocational rehabilitation agencies to help handicapped persons become employable by providing a wide range of services, financial assistance, and training. Expenses borne by the program vary according to state resources and guidelines and the recommendations of vocational rehabilitation counselors and administrators.

An individualized plan for rehabilitation is worked out with every eligible handicapped individual. The plan may include a variety of services including: a medical examination, counseling and guidance, medical help, job training, educational opportunities (including payment of college tuition), financial assistance during the rehabilitation period, referral, and job placement. If needed, on-the-job help may be extended, including travel expenses to and from work.

The federal government provides extensive support to the states for vocational rehabilitation services. The services are highly individualized, and information useful to the individual is best sought at the state or local, rather than the federal, level.

EDUCATION

The school represents one of the most effective case-finding sources for epilepsy, particularly since in the majority of cases epilepsy manifests itself during childhood. However, educational programs have not been universally responsive to the child with epilepsy. In fact, school problems often occur because of lack of understanding and recognition of the medical and psychosocial problems that epilepsy may pose for the child. Children with absence seizures are at times classified as daydreamers or inattentive. Adjustment and learning problems in children with epilepsy are not uncommon and often stem from psychological and behavior problems associated with epilepsy (see Chapter 7).

Education for All Handicapped Children Act of 1975

All children living in the United States who are between the ages of 3 and 21 and who are termed "handicapped"* are required to be served under the provisions of the Education for All Handicapped Children Act of 1975 (P.L. 93-142). The passage of this legislation reflects a movement to develop programs designed to meet each handicapped child's unique education needs. Each state is required to initiate a *Project Child Find* to locate all disabled children and youth, ages 6 to 17, and to furnish their education at public expense. Aimed to promote "mainstreaming," this law mandates that disabled children are to be identified and educated along with the nondisabled. All parents have the right to participate in and approve the individual education plan developed for their child. When children are placed in private schools by state or local educational systems in order to receive an appropriate education, this must be done at no cost to the parents. Additional services such as transportation and special aids and health-related services must also be provided at public expense.

---

*According to P.L. 94-142, Section 602, "Handicapped children" are defined as "mentally retarded, hard of hearing, deaf, speech impaired, visually handicapped, seriously emotionally disturbed, orthopedically impaired, or other health impaired, or children with specific learning disabilities, who by reason thereof require special education and related services."

According to sub-section 121a.5 (7), "other health impaired" means limited strength, vitality or alertness, due to chronic or acute health problems such as a heart condition, tuberculosis, rheumatic fever, nephritis, asthma, sickle cell anemia, hemophilia, epilepsy, lead poisoning, leukemia, or diabetes, which adversely affects a child's educational performance."

Final responsibility for implementing the federal Education for All Handicapped Children Act rests primarily with the individual state. This law is generally carried out by state departments of education, and is often delegated to special education divisions within the state department. Some states have taken the initiative to extend the federal provisions beyond the stipulated mandate provided by P.L. 94-142.

Additional information on general advocacy programs in the educational field is available from the Washington, D.C., offices of Closer Look and the Epilepsy Foundation of America.

Head Start

The 1972 Amendments to the Economic Opportunity Act call for at least 10 percent of the nationwide enrollment in Head Start to consist of children who are handicapped and require special services.

Head Start is a child development program that provides comprehensive educational and social services, parent involvement and health services to preschool children, age 3 to 5, of low-income families. More information may be available at local school boards or with Project Head Start, listed in the telephone directory.

Federal Student Financial Aid

There is no specific federal financial aid program which enables handicapped individuals to attend college, except as part of a vocational rehabilitation program. There are, however, four kinds of federal financial aid programs available to all students in need:
1. Grants given on the basis of financial need. (Money received under this condition does not have to be repaid.)
2. Loans which must be repaid.
3. Work-study programs in which a part-time job is made available.
4. Benefits, such as the GI Bill, Social Security, and Junior GI, which do not have to be repaid.

More information is available through high school guidance counselor or college financial aid offices, or by writing directly to the Bureau of Student Financial Assistance.

Vocational Education

Since 1968, a Congressional amendment to the 1963 Vocational Education Act (VEA) has mandated that 10 percent of each state's basic grant for vocational education be used exclusively to finance programs for "handicapped persons," who, because of their handicapping condition, cannot succeed without special educational assistance or a modified education program. This legislation includes persons with epilepsy, and, unlike many other educational programs which are designed exclusively for children, this program is also available for eligible handicapped adults.

Individuals eligible as "handicapped" under the Vocational Education Act are those who meet the definition of "handicapped" under the Education for All Handicapped Children Act as amended (see page 231).

An additional 10 percent for vocational education was mandated under the 1976 amendments to the Vocational Education Act, which specified that states receiving federal funds must use at least 20 percent of their funds from the federal formula grants to support vocational development guidance and counseling programs.

In order to obtain and continue to receive funds, a state is required to submit a series of documents to the United States Commissioner of Education, which specifies that current and projected programs are in compliance with federal regulations. Individuals who wish to participate in any of the vocational education programs funded under VEA basic grants are advised to apply directly to the local education agencies (LEA) or a postsecondary educational institution providing this service or administering the program.

HOUSING AND LIVING ARRANGEMENTS

In accordance with the Congressional mandate that all persons, regardless of handicap, should have the right to live within "the least restrictive environment possible," a relatively small percent of persons with the condition of "epilepsy only" are currently in institutions. According to a State Survey conducted in 1976, approximately 10 percent of residents in mental institutions and about 30 percent in institutions for the mentally retarded were reported as having seizures.

An estimated 200,000-300,000 persons with epilepsy are handicapped to the extent that they require supervised living arrangements. For this population, the development of a full spectrum of medical and social services is essential. At present, accommodations for a full range of living options for people with epilepsy who have differential needs is lacking.

Some persons could remain in a family or foster home if a daytime activity center or sheltered work program were available. An example of a day-care program for persons whose condition does not permit regular employment is conducted by the Nassau Foundation of Nassau County, New York. This day-care program offers opportunities for socialization, individual and group therapy, occupational and group therapy and rehabilitation.[5]

A wide variety of living facilities is listed in the *Guide to Epilepsy Services*, published by the Epilepsy Foundation of America.[6] Living plans vary from independent living to intermediate care facilities, and from supervised group homes to semi-independent arrangements. The reality is that the full range of differential housing and living arrangements is often difficult to locate in a community.

At the federal level, the Department of Housing and Urban Development (HUD) is responsible for the programs associated with the Housing and Community Development Act of 1974 (P.L. 93-383). Under this act, a new office of Independent Living for the Disabled has been established to promote better housing arrangements leading toward greater independence.

Group Homes

Some local and state epilepsy societies are establishing group homes where persons with epilepsy can live in a supportive setting and learn independent living skills such as cooking and housekeeping (see Chapter 8). Usually the persons accepted as residents must be employed or enrolled in a vocational training program. Most often the programs are for young adults. Since the goals of the group home programs are to prepare people for independent living, the residency period is usually limited.

Group homes for persons with epilepsy include Cincinnati's "Launching Pad," sponsored by the Greater Cincinnati Council for Epilepsy; a home in Minneapolis sponsored by the Minnesota Epilepsy League, Inc.; and homes in Farmingdale, Hicksville, and West Hempstead, New York, sponsored by the Epilepsy Foundation of Nassau County. In Cleveland, the Northeast Ohio Chapter of the Epilepsy Foundation of America sponsors a group home together with United Cerebral Palsy.

To find out whether there are plans for a group home in your community, contact the local chapter or national office of the Epilepsy Foundation of America.

Rent Subsidies

A provision of the 1974 Act for Housing and Community Development (HUD) provides rent subsidies for persons with low incomes and low interest loans for the elderly and the handicapped.

Payments by HUD are made directly to the owners of rental units to make up the difference between the HUD-approved rental amount and the amount the tenant is required to pay. Rental assistance payments under this arrangement are not considered additional income to the tenant who is also eligible for Supplemental Security Income payments from the Social Security Administration.

Requests for further information on rent assistance or other housing programs benefiting the handicapped are to be directed to the Office of Independent Living, United States Department of HUD, and/or local housing authorities.

Housing Loans

If a handicapped individual needs to remove hazards or inconvenient features in his or her home for safety reasons to make special accommodations, a Federal Housing Administration (FHA)-insured loan can be procured, up to a maximum of $10,000 per home or $5,000 per apartment unit.

Loans are applied for through banks or other financial lending institutions, and the FHA insures the lender against possible loss.

It should also be noted that individuals with low incomes may be eligible for loans from the Farmers Home Administration, through the Department of Agriculture, to purchase or repair a home that is on a farm or in a very rural area.

RESPITE SERVICES

The Plan for Nationwide Action on Epilepsy also documents a further need in the development of community-based services—namely, short-term and long-term respite care programs. These programs are meant to provide relief for parents and others responsible for the supervision of persons with uncontrolled seizures. It has been reported that even finding baby-sitters for the care of a child with epilepsy can be difficult.[7] For such services, reliance on a close acquaintance in the local community who is willing and able to accept this responsibility of child care may be the most likely resource.

TRANSPORTATION AND LICENSING

Persons with epilepsy who are not able to drive are among the "transportation disadvantaged" who are subject to restricted mobility and limited opportunities for jobs and social activities. Not having a driver's license, often a means for identification, may be an ego-deflating experience, particularly for the teenage would-be driver with epilepsy.

Driver's Licensing

Driver's licensing regulations vary considerably from state to state. Most states, however, require a documented seizure-free period, and nine states have statutes that require an individual with epilepsy be reported to a state agency, usually to the Department of Motor Vehicles.

It is generally considered preferable for the person with epilepsy rather than the physician to report to the Department of Motor Vehicles. Otherwise, the individual may not seek medical care, lest the condition be reported; and the privileged nature of the physician-patient relationship may be violated.[8]

Other Modes of Transportation

In recent years, the federal government has stepped up its efforts to make transportation systems more accessible to handicapped travelers. New regulations have been passed, and better information is now available to assist handicapped individuals in planning trips, using public transportation systems, and traveling by air, train, and bus.

Air. A publication called *Travel Tips for the Handicapped* contains the addresses of all United States airlines as well as helpful information on all modes of transportation. It is available from Consumer Information Center in Pueblo, Colorado. Another helpful publication is *Access Travel: A Guide to Accessibility of Airport Terminals*, available from Architectural & Transportation Barriers Compliance Board in Washington, D.C.

Train. Amtrak publishes a brochure, "Access Amtrak," for handicapped travelers. It can be ordered from Amtrak Public Affairs in Washington, D.C.

Toll-free information on accessibility of trains and stations and assistance available to handicapped passengers can be obtained by calling 800/523-5720, and asking for the "Special Movements Desk."

Bus. Trip information on bus rest stops and accessibility of terminals is available by inquiring at the local Greyhound or Trailways bus offices.

Access Guides

The President's Committee on Employment of the Handicapped has compiled a list of places which are accessible to people in wheelchairs or with limited mobility. Places to stay, eat, visit, or tour are included. This information is available upon request to the President's Committee.

PERSONAL SOCIAL SERVICES

The literature on epilepsy makes frequent reference to "the least understood and most neglected aspects of care—namely the social, psychological and behavioral problems."[9] These problems apparently occur as a consequence or concomitant factor associated with epilepsy. Therefore, in order to improve the social adjustment and mental health of individuals and families involved with epilepsy, a range of personal social services has been developed in mental health agencies and in general social service agencies within the public and voluntary sectors, including organized I & R programs and services.

Community Mental Health Centers (CMHC)

There are over 600 CMHCs throughout the United States. They are charged to provide services to any individual, living or employed in a defined catchment area, regardless of ability to pay, and regardless of any current or past health condition. Payment is generally determined on a sliding-fee scale.

Under the Community Mental Health Centers Act (P.L. 94-63), psychological, psychiatric, and social work services are made available to people with epilepsy "regardless of a previous health condition." A health status examination is provided as part of the initial work-up for each patient. The mental health support system is also obliged to establish liaison with other community health and social agencies, to provide consultation and education services requested by the community, and to assist in the dissemination of knowledge.

Title XX Programs

The philosophy of Title XX is to assist clients in reaching the most appropriate goal among the following: self-support, self-sufficiency, protection from abuse and neglect, community-based care, and/or institutional care.

Title XX benefits individuals with epilepsy by authorizing funds for state social service agencies to purchase or directly provide services. States have wide latitude to select which services they will provide. The range includes adoption counseling, day care, employment related, information and referral, protective, transportation, and many more specialized services. In addition, Title XX authorizes 75 percent matching money to support the training of professionals who provide services to persons with epilepsy under the States Annual Plan.

Title XX is strictly a social services program, which permits purchase of service contracts with voluntary and private agencies. Because local and state planning is required, the opportunity to participate in this planning process on behalf of epilepsy is provided.

The designation of Information and Referral Services (I & R) as a basic service under Title XX legislation is a major breakthrough, since it provides I & R services for all citizens, regardless of income, age, or residence. A growing number of states have already established or are projecting I & R networks, which are either state-administered or operate under a "contract for services" with voluntary agencies.[10]

RIGHTS, MANDATES, AND LIMITATIONS

While some of the legislated programs for services to the handicapped, such as the Vocational Rehabilitation program and the United States Employment Service, have been operating for many years, the majority of the mandated programs belong to the decade of the '70s, which Lilly Bruck has called "the Decade of Disability."[11] The newer legislation on rights for the handicapped focuses more directly on the needs of the individual handicapped person. Not only is there greater specificity, but also a mandate for case-finding through intensive and continuing efforts to locate and identify persons with handicaps and to evaluate their needs within a system of accountability.

The Developmentally-Disabled Assistance and Bill of Rights Act

The Developmentally-Disabled Assistance and Bill of Rights Act is viewed as the broadest and strongest in the series of legislative acts concerning the rights of the developmentally disabled.

In October, 1970, the first federal developmental disabilities legislation was signed into law by President Richard M. Nixon. Known as the Developmental Disabilities Services and Facilities Construction Act of 1970 (P.L. 91-517), this legislation brought under one umbrella three major disability groups (mental retardation, cerebral palsy, and epilepsy), and theoretically all other disabilities which share common service needs. The Act was amended in 1975 with the passage of the Developmentally-Disabled Assistance and Bill of Rights Act (P.L. 94-103). The 1975 amendments retained the requirements that the disability originate prior to age 18, be a substantial handicap, and continue for a lifetime. Autism was added to the list of disabilities as was dyslexia, the latter only if it was attributable to mental retardation, cerebral palsy, epilepsy or autism.

The new Developmental Disabilities Law (P.L. 95-602) passed by Congress in 1978 amends and extends the existing Developmental Disabilities Assistance and Bill of Rights Act. The new law has introduced some major new programs and made substantial changes in certain existing programs. The Congress adopted a new "functional" definition of developmental disability to replace the categorical listing (epilepsy, autism, cerebral palsy, mental retardation) found in the previous laws. The new definition states:

The term "developmental disability" means a severe, chronic disability of a person which—

(A) is attributable to a mental or physical impairment or combination of mental and physical impairments;

(B) is manifested before the person attains age twenty-two;

(C) is likely to continue indefinitely;

(D) results in substantial functional limitations in three or more of the following areas of major life activity:

(i) self-care, (ii) receptive and expressive language, (iii) learning, (iv) mobility, (v) self-direction, (vi) capacity for independent living, (vii) economic sufficiency; and

(E) reflects the person's need for a combination and sequence of special interdisciplinary, or generic care, treatment or other services which are of lifelong or extended duration and are individually planned and coordinated.

The 1978 Amendments also designate certain services as priorities for funding, recognizing that such services are of paramount importance to the severely disabled. Priority services include:

Case Management. Access to needed services, follow-through, and co-ordination services.

Child Development. Early intervention, prevention, diagnosis and evaluation.

Alternative Living Arrangement Services. Services to assist developmentally disabled persons to maintain residential arrangements in the community.

Non-vocational Social Development Services. Assists developmentally disabled persons with the performance of daily living skills.

A review of the above definitions of developmental disability and priority services indicates that the intent of the legislation is to serve those persons most in need of services; those whose epilepsy is so disabling that they cannot function adequately in one or more of life's major activities. Clearly, the definition of developmental disability does not apply to persons with epilepsy for whom the disorder of epilepsy represents only a minor life disturbance.

A major feature of the legislation is the important role of "protection and advocacy" for the rights of the developmentally disabled. A strong regulatory measure of the law is that any state failing to have a system for "protection and advocacy" may become ineligible for funding through its Developmental Disability formula grant allotment.

The Rehabilitation Act of 1973

Though rights are assured by laws, many people with epilepsy face various forms of discrimination which limit maximum independence and self-actualization.

Title V of the Rehabilitation Act of 1973, amended by the Comprehensive Rehabilitation Act of 1978, includes several provisions to eliminate discrimination towards the handicapped, including persons with epilepsy. Section 501 prevents discrimination and mandates affirmative action in federal employment; Section 502 is designed to eliminate architectural barriers; Section 503 covers discriminatory employment practices and mandated affirmative action by federal contractors; and Section 504 prohibits discriminatory practices against the handicapped in any programs or activities receiving federal financial assistance. Since 1978, Section 504 also applies to all federal agencies. It is broader than any other prior legislation, since it covers all kinds of discrimination, over and beyond employment. In the event complaints are made relevant to Section 504, grievance procedures are carried out by the Office for Civil Rights.

LEGAL ASSISTANCE SERVICES

One avenue of legal assistance is the Legal Services Corporation which is a private, non-profit organization created and funded by Congress to provide legal assistance in civil matters to people with low incomes. Each local program sets its own financial eligibility standards, taking local living costs into account. Other avenues of legal assistance include recourse to "the protection and advocacy system" available in each state, bar association projects, public interest law projects, and local advocacy groups.

RESOURCES FOR INFORMATION AND SERVICES

To date there is no general data base on information for the handicapped person, and no integrated formal network of groups and agencies providing information on services and advocacy for the handicapped, including epilepsy. There is, however, general agreement that an Information and Referral (I & R) service should be a universal doorway to available resources, offered free of charge, and aimed to promote access through an organized, updated, and retrievable information system.

Essential functions of an I & R program include information-giving, advice, referral, and adequate follow-up to insure accountability. Concrete services such as transportation and escort services may be provided. Levels of counseling and the extent of advocacy depend upon the agency's mission, level of funding, and staffing patterns.[12]

Federal Resources

The Office for Handicapped Individuals (OHI) within the Office of Human Development (OHD) collects and disseminates a variety of information materials on handicapped persons, including those with epilepsy. The national Clearinghouse in OHI seeks to improve the lives of handicapped individuals by enhancing the flow of information through its publications. The Clearinghouse also responds to inquiries from handicapped individuals and serves as a resource to organizations involved in programs relevant to the handicapped.[13]

According to an OHI report, there are more than 20 national directories on the handicapped that list services or organizations by state. The latest *Directory of Information Sources on Handicapping Conditions and Related Services* lists a broad range of national organizations and federal information sources. *Federal Assistance for Programs Serving the Handicapped* was published by OHI in 1976. A series of booklets, published by the Federal Programs Information and Assistance Project, describes federal resources to assist developmentally disabled people.

To disseminate biomedical research for the general public, the National Institute of Neurological and Communicative Disorders and Stroke (NINCDS) provides information through its "Hope Through Research" series of pamphlets.

State Programs

There is great variability in the availability of information on a state level, particularly since few states have a reasonably complete inventory of services for the disabled. It is important for information providers to know that some specialized services and resources may only exist in one or a few locations in a state (or region).

The agency names and range of services for the many health and social service organizations which assume specific areas of responsibility on a state level vary from state to state, and some types of services may be included in some State Offices for Mental Retardation, State Crippled Children's Services, or State Vocational Rehabilitation Offices that do not exist in other state offices of a like name.

With the support of Title XX funds, a growing number of states are beginning to develop state-wide I & R systems. Some operate with a centralized, toll-free line, others by networking local I & R programs; some use a combination of both.[14] The United States Administration on Aging promotes a vigorous I & R program in state and area agencies.[15]

Local Services

Local information resources are often difficult to locate, yet this is the most crucial level at which service delivery for the person with epilepsy takes place.

The yellow pages of the local telephone directory are not to be underestimated for listings of agencies. A likely initial contact would be inquiry at an Information and Referral Service which might be operating in a municipal office, in a local library, or in a Health and Welfare Council.[16] (The United Way has been a forerunner in the development of I & R Services within Community Councils.) More specifically concerned with services for handicapped persons are Easter Seal Society Information IR & F Centers (Information, Referral, and Follow-Up), which are located in some 207 sites across the country.

Libraries have developed special services for handicapped persons and are becoming increasingly and more dynamically involved in the operation and delivery of I & R Services.[17] Some municipal governments are developing advocacy programs, including hot-lines, crisis lines, and information centers for handicapped persons. For example, the New York City Mayor's Office provides an I & R Service for the disabled.

It is also likely that the local chapter of the national Epilepsy Foundation of America will be most helpful to the person with epilepsy in need of information, services, and continued assistance.

The Voluntary Sector

Epilepsy Foundation of America (EFA). The unification of three national voluntary agencies into a single organization, the Epilepsy Foundation of America (EFA), has mobilized a stronger movement for epilepsy than has ever existed before. This nationwide organization functions at national, state, and local levels. As of 1980, EFA reported 50 affiliated chapters, 23 provisional chapters, and 105 information contacts.[18]

On a national level, EFA is the spokesman and advocate for the rights of persons with epilepsy. Planning, policy formulation, I & R, fundraising, and coordinating resources for epilepsy also occur on a state level. Direct services are provided by staff of local EFA chapters, and include information dissemination and referrals, training programs, and public education, as well as sponsorship of self-help groups. Extensive EFA publications include free pamphlets, lists of books, directories, films, and visual aids. *Basic Statistics for the Epilepsies,* as well as a *Guide to Epilepsy Services,* are major publications of the EFA.

Alliance of Information and Referral Services (AIRS). A notable development in promoting systematized access to available services has been the organization of the National Alliance of Information and Referral Services (AIRS). Formally organized in 1972, AIRS has sought to develop standards, establish criteria, and promote communication and coordination amongst the providers of I & R programs in the public and voluntary sectors, including organizations which serve the handicapped.

AIRS publishes a newsletter, a professional quarterly, a *Directory of I & R Services in the United States and Canada,* and Standards for I & R Services. The *Directory* lists a total of over 600 I & R programs under public and voluntary auspices, including I & R services mandated by the Administration on Aging for all AOA state and area agencies.

Other Voluntary Agencies. Other health organizations which operate direct I & R services as well as training programs for local I & R providers include the Easter Seals for Crippled Children and Adults, and the American Red Cross. A variety of local volunteer groups, such as church-based and special interest groups, have organized I & R services for selected age groups and around specific problems such as alcoholism and drug abuse. Hot-lines have sprung up overnight to provide peer counseling, especially for youth involved in crisis problems. Newspapers, radio, and television programs have established I & R-type programs, such as the popular "Call for Action" programs.

RECOMMENDATIONS

While there are many sources of information, expanding numbers of human service agencies, and increased legislative mandates to improve the lives of the handicapped, many persons with epilepsy remain unserved or underserved. For many, a great deal of pathology could be prevented through early and systematic access to services.

Up to this point, the discussion has dealt primarily with substantive information and reported data on resources for epilepsy. However, it is the translation and application of this knowledge into a process of linking consumer and resource that actualizes access. This process is a primary responsibility of the service provider.

The process of monitoring the client from the point of inquiry or entry to the point of service completion is indeed complex, and often frustrating.

Skills and expertise, as well as knowledge of resources, are required on the part of the service provider. Acquiring information, processing referrals, and conducting advocacy programs are not discrete components, but rather represent interrelated elements within a viable system of Information Referral and Advocacy (IRA)[19] These relationships are illustrated in Figure 1.

Information Acquisition

Information tasks include a basic knowledge of the disorder of epilepsy and an understanding of the specific concerns of the individual and family involved in epilepsy. Analysis of relevant legislation and a working knowledge of the services available on local, state, and federal levels are aspects of the information armamentarium which providers need to possess.

Given the enormous volume and diversity of service organizations, facilities, and programs, a system for the organization of a resource file would be advisable, with capabilities for update and ease in retrieval. While most resource files of local agencies may now rely on manual card systems, a knowledge of automated human services systems, which have proliferated during the past decade, is essential. The technology of information systems and electric data processing are invaluable tools in the organization and maintenance of resource data.

A responsible reporting system which documents the incidence and prevalence of epilepsy in a particular area is fundamental to an I & R operation. The compiled data represent a valuable fund of community information, and could be very helpful in community planning. In fact, the planning function of I & R systems is increasingly recognized to be of equal importance to the service functions of an I & R system.[20]

Referral Process

The heart of the IRA System is the referral system that includes a continuum of information-giving, from simple inquiries (for example, the hours of the seizure clinic) to far more complex situations (such as arrangements for an independent living plan). It is generally helpful to view the I & R functions as a spectrum of services, which ranges from "information only" to advice and counseling, with provision for treatment as may be diagnostically determined.

Referral without follow-up can be of very limited usefulness. Selective or universal follow-up would be a matter of professional judgment as well as agency policy, and might also follow a continuum. A simple follow-up would be to ascertain whether or not the consumer reached the agency. A more

Figure 1

An Access System—IRA
Access to Resources for Epilepsy

Information Acquisition	Referral Process	Advocacy Action
Knowledge —of Epilepsy —of relevant legislation —of services available on federal, state and local levels	Counseling——Treatment Follow-Up——Follow-Through	Assertion of Consumer Rights Utilization of Legal Remedies Negotiation with Service Systems Promotion of Community Action Groups
The Resource File —organization and maintenance —update and retrieval	Agency Action to Inter-agency Activities	Support of Self-Help Groups Outreach to unserved and potential consumers
Reporting System —Service Statistics —Planning Data		Education, Training, Research

complex follow-up or follow-through would be to establish whether the service was given, and to assess what was the outcome.

By definition, an I & R system is an interagency operation which needs to develop an infrastructure based on interorganizational associations and collaborations.

Advocacy Action

Advocacy fosters self-initiative, independence and the utilization of resources by the person directly involved with epilepsy. Although the primary definition of an advocate is "one who pleads the cause of another," the following advocacy strategies broaden this definition to include not only single case advocacy, but also systems or policy advocacy, self-help or consumer advocacy, and legal advocacy.

The assumption underlying case advocacy is that the persons are impaired to the extent that either volunteer-citizens or professionals are needed to represent the interests of the disabled and to promote their cause. Rather than meeting the needs of disabled individuals, systems or policy advocacy implies working as a group or coalition to change laws or policies or to develop new programs.

The promotion of self-help or consumer advocacy activities has demonstrated the effectiveness of self-help groups in carrying out dynamic advocacy programs, as well as in serving the mutual aid and personal interests of the individual group members.[21] Experience in self-help advocacy has indicated that "being involved in determining one's own destiny provides a sense of self-worth and belonging, and reduces feelings of isolation and withdrawal.[22] Based on the premise that persons with epilepsy have the right, and therefore should have the opportunity, to promote their own well-being, the Epilepsy Foundation of America's federally funded Self-Help or Consumer Advocacy Project has been established to enable viable, self-standing consumer groups to participate in service planning and to impact upon service delivery.

Legal advocacy implies the use of litigation to ensure and protect the rights of handicapped persons. As noted earlier, the Developmentally Disabled Assistance and Bill of Rights Act (P.L. 94-103) established statutory mechanisms to protect the rights of persons with developmental disabilities. This act stipulates that each state must have a legal advocacy program "to protect and advocate" for the rights of the disabled who are receiving treatment, services, or rehabilitation.

With the support of developmental disabilities legislation, the major thrust in advocacy efforts has been by non-profit voluntary organizations.[23] The

Epilepsy Foundation of America and its local chapters, and other non-affiliated organizations, such as the Epilepsy Center of Michigan, promote a variety of advocacy programs which represent one or more of the four advocacy approaches discussed above—case and policy advocacy, self-help and legal advocacy. Vital to any effective advocacy program is a strong emphasis on educational and training opportunities for consumers as well as providers of services.

A Comprehensive Epilepsy Service Network (CESN)

In spite of the broad and multitudinous array of health and social service organizations, no mechanism currently exists for coordinating service or providing the comprehensive care needed by persons with epilepsy. To provide a viable and responsive service network accessible to individuals with epilepsy and their families, the Commission for the Control of Epilepsy and Its Consequences has suggested a Comprehensive Epilepsy Service Network (CESN). As noted in Figure 2, this Network design includes the following four major components:

Existing Community Service Providers: General health and social service agencies.

Community Resource Persons: A specialist in information and referral services, training and resource development.

Epilepsy Family and Individual Resource Teams: Interdisciplinary teams which will provide back-up support to the community providers on special problems, provide specialized medical and social services, and outreach capability for training and counseling.

An Office for Special Neurological Impairments: At the federal level, a unit to assume responsibility for the placement of Community Resource Persons and Epilepsy Family and Individual Resource Teams for guiding public and professional education, resource development and quality content, standard setting and evaluation.

With a view toward optimizing existing resources, the Commission has recommended that Information and Referral services be made available through access to central resource directories, since "knowing where and how to get service is a key factor in prevention and treatment".[24]

Until such time that viable and comprehensive service networks will be developed to facilitate improved access to services for persons with epilepsy, providers of services will need to develop effective linkages with needed

Figure 2

Comprehensive Epilepsy Service Network

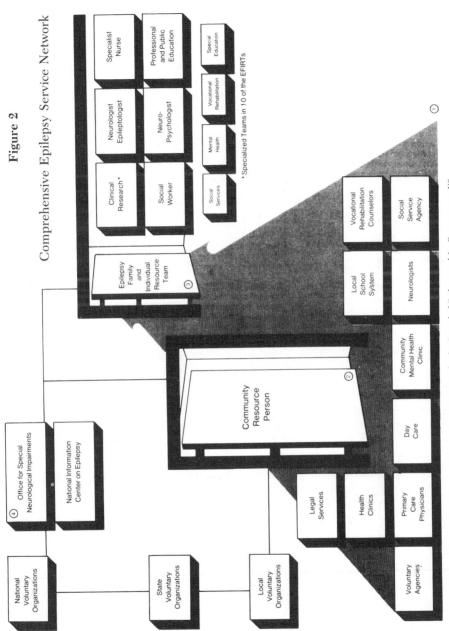

Source: *Plan for Nationwide Action on Epilepsy*, The Commission for the Control of Epilepsy and Its Consequences. US DHEW, Volume I, p. 151.

resources. Training for professionals, paraprofessionals, and volunteers is essential for informed providers in the field of epilepsy. Public education programs are indispensable for informed consumers.

Until social research in epilepsy is expanded to include more experimentation and testing of service delivery systems and modes of improved access, providers of services must continue to rely on their own resourcefulness with resources.

DIRECTORY OF SELECTED SERVICES

Medical and Dental Care and Medical Assistance

1. American Medical Association (AMA)
   535 North Dearborn Street
   Chicago, Illinois 60610
2. American Dental Association and
   Academy of Dentistry for the Handicapped
   211 E. Chicago Avenue
   Chicago, Illinois 60611
3. Health Care Financing Administration
   Medicare Bureau, Health Education Inquiries Branch
   Lowrise, Room GB3
   Baltimore, Maryland 21235
4. Health Financing Administration
   Medical Services Administration
   Social & Rehabilitation Service
   U.S. Dept. of Health, Education, and Welfare (HEW)
   Washington, D.C.
5. EFA Low-Cost Drug Program
   % Prescription Delivery Service
   126 South York Road
   Hatboro, Pennsylvania 19040
6. Tel-Med., Inc.
   National Headquarters
   P.O. Box 5249
   San Bernardino, California 92412

Insurance

EFA Insurance—Group Life Plan
Epilepsy Foundation of America
1828 L. Street, N.W.
Washington, D.C. 20036

Tax Benefits

>   U.S. Internal Revenue Service (IRS)
>   Washington, D.C.

Employment and Vocational Rehabilitation

1. *Working Together . . . The Key to Jobs for the Handicapped. An AFL-CIO Guide*
   AFL-CIO
   815 Sixteenth Street, N.W.
   Washington, D.C. 20036
2. Interagency Committee on Employment of the Handicapped
   Civil Service Commission
   1900 E. Street, N.W.
   Washington, D.C. 20415
3. Office of Federal Contracts Compliance Programs
   Department of Labor
   600 D. Street, S.W.
   Washington, D.C. 20201
4. The Disability Rights Center
   1346 Connecticut Avenue
   Washington, D.C. 20036
5. Federal Information Centers
   General Services Administration
   Washington, D.C. 20405
6. National Clearinghouse of Rehabilitation Training Materials
   Oklahoma State University
   115 Old USDA Building
   Stillwater, Oklahoma 74074
7. Office for Civil Rights
   Department of Health, Education, and Welfare
   300 Independence Avenue, S.W.
   Washington, D.C. 20201
8. President's Committee on Employment of the Handicapped
   Department of Labor
   1111-20th Street, N.W.
   Washington, D.C. 20210
9. Small Business Administration
   Director, Office of Financing
   1441 L. Street, N.W.
   Washington, D.C. 20416

Education

1. Bureau of Education for the Handicapped
   U.S. Office of Education
   400 Maryland Avenue, S.W.
   Washington, D.C. 20202
2. Bureau of Student Financial Assistance
   P.O. Box 84
   Washington, D.C. 20044
3. Closer Look
   National Information Center
   P.O. Box 1492
   Washington, D.C. 20013
4. Council for Exceptional Children
   CEC Information Services
   1920 Association Drive
   Reston, Virginia
5. Headstart
   Office of Child Development
   Office for Human Development Services
   Department of Health, Education, and Welfare
   Washington, D.C. 20201
6. Information Center for Handicapped Children
   1619 M. Street, N.W.
   Washington, D.C. 20036

Housing and Living Arrangements

1. Farmers Home Administration
   Department of Agriculture
   Washington, D.C. 20250
2. National Association of Housing and Redevelopment Officials
   2600 Virginia Avenue, N.W.
   Washington, D.C. 20037
3. United States Department of Housing and Urban Development
   Washington, D.C. 20410
4. United States Department of Housing and Urban Development
   HUD's Office for Independent Living for the Disabled
   7th Street and D. Street, S.W.
   Washington, D.C. 20410

5. Group homes:
   Epilepsy Foundation of America, Inc.
   1828 L. Street, N.W., Suite 406
   Washington, D.C. 20036
   Or local epilepsy society

Transportation and Licensing

1. Amtrak Public Affairs
   955 L'Enfant Plaza, S.W.
   Washington, D.C. 20024
2. Architectural and Transportation Barriers Compliance Board
   Washington, D.C. 20201
3. Consumer Information Center
   Pueblo, Colorado 81009

Personal Social Services

American Alliance for Health, Physical Education and
   Recreation
1201 16th Street, N.W.
Washington, D.C. 20036

*Organizations Involved in Information, Referral, and
Advocacy for Epilepsy*

1. Alliance of Information and Referral Services
   P.O. Box 10705
   Phoenix, Arizona 85064
2. American Association of University-Affiliated Programs for the
   Developmentally Disabled
   1100 17th Street, N.W.
   Suite 908
   Washington, D.C. 20036
3. Clearinghouse on the Handicapped
   Office for Handicapped Individuals
   Office of Human Development
   Department of Health, Education, and Welfare
   339-South Portal Bldg.
   200 Independence Avenue, S.W.
   Washington, D.C. 20201

4. Consumer Information Center
   Pueblo, Colorado 81009
5. Epilepsy Foundation of America, Inc.
   1828 L Street, N.W., Suite 406
   Washington, D.C. 20036
6. Epilepsy International
   2 bis, chemin Auguste-Vilbert
   1218 Grand Saconnen
   Geneva, Switzerland
7. International Bureau for Epilepsy
   2 bis, chemin Auguste-Vilbert
   1218 Grand Saconnen
   Geneva, Switzerland
8. National Association of Epilepsy Executives
   P.O. Box 2572
   Houston, Texas 77005
9. National Center for Law and the Handicapped
   1235 N. Eddy Street
   South Bend, Indiana 46617
10. National Easter Seal Society for Crippled Children and Adults
    2023 West Ogden Avenue
    Chicago, Illinois 60612
11. National Epilepsy League
    6 North Michigan Avenue
    Chicago, Illinois 60602
12. National Institute of Neurological and Communicative Disorders
    and Stroke
    National Institutes of Health
    Public Health Service
    Department of Health, Education, and Welfare
    Building 31
    Bethesda, Maryland 20014
13. International League Against Epilepsy
    2 bis, chemin Auguste-Vilbert
    1218 Grand Saconnen
    Geneva, Switzerland
14. Rehabilitation International U.S.A.
    20 W. 40th Street
    New York, New York 10018

RESOURCE READINGS

Background Information

Parsonage, M. J. (ed.) *Prevention of Epilepsy and its Consequences*. London: International Bureau for Epilepsy, 1973.

Sands, Harry and Minters, Frances C. *The Epilepsy Fact Book*. F. A. Davis Company, 1977; Charles Scribner's Sons, 1979.

Scott, Donald F. *About Epilepsy*. (Revised ed.), New York: International Universities, 1973.

Silverstein, Alvin and Silverstein, Virginia B. *Epilepsy*. Philadelphia, Pennsylvania: I. B. Lippincott & Co. 1975.

Temkin, Oswei. *The Falling Sickness: A History of Epilepsy from the Greeks to the Beginnings of Modern Neurology*. Baltimore: John Hopkins Press, 1971.

Volle, Frank O. and Heron, Patricia, A. *Epilepsy and You*. Springfield, Illinois: Charles C. Thomas, 1978.

Wright, George N. (ed.) *Epilepsy Rehabilitation*. Boston, Mass: Little, Brown & Co. 1975.

Children and Youth

Bagley, Christopher, *The Social Psychology of the Epileptic Child*. Coral Gables, Fla: University of Miami Press, 1971.

Baird, Henry W., *The Child with Convulsions: A Guide for Parents, Teachers, Counselors, and Medical Personnel*. New York: Grune & Stratton, 1972.

Goldin, George J., *The Rehabilitation of the Young Epileptic*. Boston, Mass: D. C. Heath & Co., 1971.

Gollay, Elinor and Bennett, Alivena, *The College Guide for Students with Disabilities*. Cambridge, Mass: Abt Publications, 55 Wheeler St., Cambridge, Mass 02138.

Kyle, Larryette M. *An Advocacy Manual for Parents of Handicapped Children*. Los Angeles, California: Institute for Child Advocacy, 1976.

Lagos, Jorge C. *Seizures, Epilepsy and Your Child*. New York: Harper & Row, 1974.

Livingston, Samuel, *Comprehensive Management of Epilepsy in Infancy, Childhood and Adolescence*. Springfield, Illinois: Charles C. Thomas, 1971.

Rights and Entitlements

Action: A Manual for Organizing and Conducting PPHC Area Meetings. Published by Parents & Professionals for Handicapped Children, Inc., Raleigh, North Carolina, 1975.

Kalbacker, David. (Epilepsy Society of Massachusetts). *How to Organize a Consumer Workshop on Epilepsy.* Washington, D.C.: Epilepsy Foundation of America, 1976.

The Legal Rights of Persons with Epilepsy. (A Survey of State Laws and Administrative Policies). Epilepsy Foundation of America, 1976 Edition.

Nalls, Jim O. and Pardue, Carolyn R. (Florida Epilepsy Foundation). *Organizational and Developmental Principles for Successful Self-Help Groups.* Washington, D.C.: The Epilepsy Foundation of America, 1976.

O'Keefe, Pat. *Helping Other Persons with Epilepsy.* Saint Paul, Minnesota: Minnesota Epilepsy League, Inc., 1976.

Your Child's Right to an Education: A Guide for Parents of Handicapped Children in New York State. The N.Y. State Education Dept. Office for Education of Children with Handicapping Conditions, 1978.

Your Rights under the Education for all Handicapped Children Act. P.L. 94-142 (March 1976). Washington, D.C.

Guides, Directories, and Plans

Boshes, Louis D. and Gibbs, Frederic A. *Epilepsy Handbook*, 2nd Edition, Springfield, Illinois: Charles C. Thomas, 1972.

Bruck, Lilly. *Access: The Guide to a Better Life for Disabled Americans.* New York: Random House, 1978.

Cereghino, James J. *Surveying Facilities Available to the Person with Epilepsy.* A 50-State Guide Developed by the Epilepsy Foundation of America, 1972.

Coleman, Jean and Levinson, Risha W. (eds.) *Directory on Resources for Information and Referral Materials*, Alliance of Information and Referral Services, 1979.

Directory of Federal Consumer Offices. Consumer Information Center, Pueblo, Colorado 81009.

Directory of National Information Sources on Handicapping Conditions and Related Services. Department of Health, Education, and Welfare: Clearinghouse on the Handicapped Office for Handicapped Individuals. First edition, December, 1976.; 2nd Edition, May, 1980.

Eckstein, Burton J. (ed.) *Handicapped Funding Directory*, 1978-79 Edition. Oceanside, N.Y.: Research Grant Guides, P.O. Box 357.

Epilepsy Foundation of America. *A Guide to Epilepsy Services.* Washington, D.C., 1978.

Federal Programs Information and Assistance Project. Washington, D.C. Bureau of Developmental Disabilities, Department of Health, Education, and Welfare:

   Modules for Technical Assistance Workshops (1976-present):
      1. Orientation to the Government Process

2. Developmental Disabilities
3. Social Services
4. Housing Development Programs
5. Intermediate Care Facilities
6. Income Maintenance
7. Planning for Action
8. Vocational Education/Vocational Rehabilitation
9. Transportation
10. Health Services
11. Employment and Training
The Guide to Federal Benefits and Programs for Handicapped Citizens and Their Families.

Gordon, Milluhop I. *A National Directory of Clinic Facilities for the Diagnosis & Treatment of Persons with Epilepsy.* Washington, D.C.: Epilepsy Foundation of America, 1973.

Insurance Handbook for Persons with Epilepsy. Washington, D.C.: Epilepsy Foundation of America.

Masland, Richard L., et al. *Plan for Nationwide Action on Epilepsy.* Report of the Commission for the Control of Epilepsy and Its Consequences. Washington, D.C.: U.S. Government Printing Office, 1977.

Penry, J. Kiffin. *Epilepsy Bibliography.* (1950-1975). Key Word & Author Indexes. U.S. Department of Health, Education, & Welfare, DHEW Publication # (NIH) 76-1186, 1976.

Schlesinger, Lawrence E. and Frank, Donald S. *Epilepsy: On the Way to Work: A Guide for the Rehabilitation Counselor.* Sponsored by the Epilepsy Foundation of America. Washington, D.C.: Arterts & Winters Syndicate, 1976.

Strudler, Lewis A. and Perlman, Leonard G. *Basic Statistics on the Epilepsies.* Prepared by the Epilepsy Foundation of America, 1828 L. Street, N.W. Washington, D.C. 20036; Philadelphia: F. A. Davis Company, 1975. (Introductory Insert.—Update, 1978).

Summary of Existing Legislation Relating to the Handicapped. Department of Education, Office of Special Education and Rehabilitative Services, Office for Handicapped Individuals. Washington, D.C., August, 1980.

Periodicals

Disabled U.S.A., President's Committee on Employment.
Epilepsia, American Epilepsy Society.
Epilepsy International Newsletter, Epilepsy International.
Information and Referral, The Journal of the Alliance of Information and Referral Systems, Inc., biannual journal.

International Rehabilitation Review, Rehabilitation International.
National News, Quarterly Publication, Epilepsy Foundation of America.
The National Spokesman, Monthly Publication of the Epilepsy Foundation of America.
Perspectives on Epilepsy, The British Epilepsy Association, annual journal.
Rehabilitation World, Rehabilitation International U.S.A.

Films and Visual Aids

Epilepsy Films and Audio Visuals (for lay and professional audiences).

A list of films and audiovisuals is available from the Epilepsy Foundation of America with information on availability and charges for materials obtained from EFA Service Centers and other suppliers.

NOTES AND REFERENCES

1. American Public Welfare Association, *Washington Report*, Volume 14, Number 1, January 1979, p. 5.
2. Levinson, R. W. Helping the needy get help—the I & R services. National Association of Social Workers *Newsletter*, 23(6):8-9, June 1978.
3. "EFA Insurance Program," Epilepsy Foundation of America, *Guide to Epilepsy Services*, March 1976, p. 120.
4. "Review of Public and Private Resources," *Plan for Nationwide Action on Epilepsy*, The Commission for the Control of Epilepsy and Its Consequences. U.S. Dept. of HEW, Public Health Service, National Institute of Health, 1977, p. 202.
5. Rosenblum, P. Epic day center expands. *Epi-Log*, Epilepsy Foundation of Nassau County, 14(1):2, May, 1979.
6. *Guide to Epilepsy Services*, op. cit., pp. 87-89.
7. *Plan for Nationwide Action on Epilepsy*, op. cit., p. 122.
8. Ibid., p. 108.
9. Ibid., p. 17; also see Chapter 3, "Living with Epilepsy" in *The Epilepsy Fact Book* by Harry Sands and Frances Minters, Philadelphia, Pennsylvania: F. A. Davis Company, 1977, pp. 43-70; also see Tony Arangio, "A Position Paper: A Systematic Examination of the Psycho-Social Needs of Patients with Epilepsy," *The Need for a Comprehensive Change Approach*, in *Plan for Nationwide Action on Epilepsy*, op. cit., Volume II, Part 1, 1977, pp. 366-387.
10. Hercenberg, J. Information and referral services funding under title XX. In: *Proceedings of the Information and Referral Roundtable*, 1976, published by Alliance of Information and Referral Services, Inc., Phoenix, Arizona, 1977, pp. 61-63.
11. Bruck, L. *Access: The Guide to a Better Life for Disabled Americans*, New York: Random House, 1978, p. 4.
12. Kahn, A. J. et al., *Neighborhood Information Center*, New York: Columbia University School of Social Work, 1966, p. 116.
13. Bruck, L., op. cit., pp. 94-95.
14. Day, S. L. The implementation of information and referral services under Title XX in Massachusetts; also, Isaacs, W. A. Title XX implementation: Information and referral services in Cleveland, Ohio; also, Norris, C. A. Title XX implementation: State of Arizona. In: *Proceedings of the Information and Referral Roundtable*, 1976, op. cit., pp. 65-95.
15. *Program Development Handbook for State and Area Agencies on Information and Referral Services for the Elderly*, published by Administration on Aging, Office of Human Development Series, U.S. Dept. of Health, Education and Welfare, Washington, D.C. 20201,

October 1977. The Administration on Aging has also organized a federal task force through working agreements with 15 governmental agency representatives to promote coordination of I & R networks on federal, state and local levels.

16. Most of the local community health and welfare councils are members of the national United Way of America. The United Way was the first national organization to develop a standardized classification system for Information and Referral Services, which is referred to as the United Way of America Service Identification System (UWASIS).

17. See M. Kochen and J. C. Donahue. *Information for the Community*, Chicago, Illinois: American Library Association, 1974; also, M. Braverman (ed.). Information and referral services in the public library. Special Edition, *Drexel Library Quarterly*, Philadelphia, PA: Drexel University, Vol. 12, Nos. 1, 2, January-April 1976.

18. Updated information provided by Nyrma Hernandez, Deputy Executive Director for Program Services, Epilepsy Foundation of America, Washington, D.C.

19. *National Standards for Information and Referral Services*, Alliance of Information and Referral Services, Phoenix, Arizona, 1978.

20. Ibid., pp. 2, 3, 5, 11.

21. Kahn, A. op. cit., p. 118.

22. O'Keefe, P. *Helping Other Persons With Epilepsy*, St. Paul, Minnesota: Epilepsy League, Inc., 1976.

23. *Plan for Nationwide Action on Epilepsy*, op. cit., p. 150.

24. *Plan for Nationwide Action on Epilepsy*, op. cit., pp. 249-330.

EPILOGUE

HARRY SANDS, PH.D.

The past decades have produced major advances in the treatment of epilepsy. Clinical and neuroscience research programs have produced antiepileptic drugs that enable 80 percent of persons with epilepsy to achieve control of their seizures with minimal or no toxic effects. Thus, attention can now be given to preventing and controlling the psychological and social factors which comprise the epilepsy syndrome. The psychosocial management of the seizure patient is essential to the treatment of the convulsive disorders. Accordingly, the mental health clinicians—psychiatrists, psychologists, social workers, psychiatric nurses, and rehabilitation and educational counselors—must work together with neurologists, electroencephalographers, and clinical neuroscientists as the providers of comprehensive management to the seizure patient. This approach, which is practiced in the federally funded comprehensive Epilepsy Centers of Excellence, needs to be extended to every clinic, mental health center, and practitioner who treats patients with epilepsy.

The psychological and the social problems are a consequence of epilepsy for all patients. As links in the behavior chain, the psychological and social interact with each other and with other links in the chain and contribute to the adjustment of the individual to the seizures and to the tasks of independent living. Comprehensive treatment of the seizure patient is based on an assessment of each link in the behavior chain. The diagnostic study determines the treatment plan that will maximize the individual's freedom from seizures and adjustment to physical and developmental deficits, and minimize the psychosocial factors that interfere with coping and adjustment. To effectively treat the epilepsy patient, mental health professionals must have a dynamic understanding of each link in the behavior chain and how it has affected the epilepsy patient. This understanding can then be used to help the patient gain understanding, and to define the treatment goals and the procedure of choice to reach them. The therapeutic alliance is then used to work through the problems; the therapist and the patient actively work together to convert the patient's insight into actions designed to change his or her behavior; that is, to cope with epilepsy and its consequences.

Clearly the seizure patient cannot be effectively treated by use of a single therapeutic modality. Anticonvulsant drugs control seizures. They do not necessarily or by themselves change the epilepsy patient's or family's, or the community's attitudes and feelings toward the epilepsy. Nor do they undo the traumatic experiences or the developmental deficits which often result from seizures. These are the psychological and social consequences of epilepsy that must be addressed by the mental health practitioner if the person with epilepsy is to have free access to the social process and to the full use of his or her abilities and capacities.

Any barrier to this access—whether the barrier comes from the patient or from the community—will result in the patient's impairment becoming a handicap. The comprehensive treatment delivery system must prevent this from happening. To achieve the elimination of barriers, members of the clinical team must go beyond the consulting room to act on behalf of the person with epilepsy. We must become active advocates, participating in social action programs of our professional and scientific societies and voluntary health organizations such as the Epilepsy Foundation of America. Only in this way will we be successful in removing specific barriers against a particular patient.

INDEX